Love Is M

There seems to be a perennial fascination with Gypsies: their lifestyles, beliefs, customs, traditions, and especially their knowledge of occult lore. To many they are workers of magick—mysterious and charming people who can "make things happen." The Gypsies are living magicians among us.

One of the most compelling forms of magick—perhaps the most sought after—is love magick. It is a *positive* form of working, a way to true delight and pleasure. The Gypsies have long been known for the successful working of love magick.

In this book you will find sections on love magick for those who are courting (The Thrill of the Chase), love magick for newlyweds (The Golden Rings), and love magick for the family unit (The Family Circle). There is also a section on Gypsy love potions, talismans, amulets, and charms.

Included are spells and charms to discover your future spouse, to make your lover your best friend, to bring love into a loveless marriage, and to cause a runaway to return home. You will learn traditional secrets gathered from English Gypsies that are presented here for the first time ever by a Gypsy of Romani blood.

Throughout the book two things are emphasized: practicality and positivity. All the magickal spells and charms can be done using ordinary, everyday items, and none of them will harm another person or interfere with another's free will.

Even if you don't intend to practice, *Secrets of Gypsy Love Magick* will entertain and enlighten you on the subject of love and Gypsies.

ABOUT THE AUTHOR

Ray Buckland's grandfather was the first of the Buckland Gypsies to give up traveling the roads in waggons and to settle in a permanent house. From his earliest years Ray remembers listening to his father's and grandfather's tales of Romani life, and watching his grandmother read cards and tell fortunes. This early upbringing instilled in him a deep respect for the Old Ways. From his teens, Ray Buckland started his own serious studies of the Old Knowledge, and later, came to write about it in a number of best-selling books. "Buckland" is a well-known name among English Gypsies, and Ray Buckland has become a well-known author of books on practical magic. He is today regarded as one of the leading authorities on witchcraft, voodoo and the supernatural.

To Write to the Author

We cannot guarantee that every letter written to the author can be answered, but all will be forwarded. Both the author and the publisher appreciate hearing from readers, learning of your enjoyment and benefit from this book. Llewellyn also publishes a bi-monthly news magazine with news and reviews of practical esoteric studies and articles helpful to the student, and some readers' questions and comments to the author may be answered through this magazine's columns if permission to do so is included in the original letter. The author sometimes participates in seminars and workshops, and dates and places are announced in *The Llewellyn New Times*. To write to the author, or to ask a question, write to:

Raymond Buckland
c/o THE LLEWELLYN NEW TIMES
P.O. Box 64383-053, St. Paul, MN 55164-0383, U.S.A.
Please enclose a self-addressed, stamped envelope for reply, or $1.00 to cover costs.

Llewellyn's New Age Series

Secrets of Gypsy Love Magick

Raymond Buckland

1994
Llewellyn Publications
St. Paul, Minnesota 55164-0383

FIRST EDITION
Fourth Printing, 1994

Cover Painting: Lissanne Lake

Library of Congress Cataloging-in-Publication Data
  Buckland, Raymond.
    Secrets of Gypsy love magick/Raymond Buckland
        p.   cm.—(Llewellyn's new age series)
ISBN 0-87542-053-2
1. Magic, Gypsy. 2. Aphrodisiacs. 3. Charms.
4. Gypsies-Social life and customs.   I. Title   II. Series
DX155.B831623.P5C86   1990
133.4'42
                                   89-77239
                                       CIP

Llewellyn Publications
A Division of Llewellyn Worldwide, Ltd.
P.O. Box 64383, St. Paul, MN 55164-0383

ABOUT LLEWELLYN'S NEW AGE SERIES

The "New Age"—it's phrase we use, but what does it mean? Does it mean that we are entering the Aquarian Age? Does it mean that a new Messiah is coming to correct all that is wrong and make Earth into a Garden? Probably not—but the idea of a *major change* is there, combined with awareness that Earth *can* be a Garden; that war, crime, poverty, disease, etc., are not necessary "evils."

Optimists, dreamers, scientists . . . nearly all of us believe in a "better tomorrow," and that somehow we can do things now that will make for a better future life for ourselves and for coming generations.

In one sense, we all know there's nothing new under the Heavens, and in another sense that every day makes a new world. The difference is in our consciousness. And this is what the New Age is all about it's a major change in consciousness found within each of us as we learn to bring forth and manifest powers that Humanity has always potentially had.

Evolution moves in "leaps." Individuals struggle to develop talents and powers, and their efforts build a "power bank" in the Collective Unconsciousness, the soul of Humanity that suddenly makes these same talents and powers easier access for the majority.

You still have to learn the "rules" for developing and applying these powes, but it is more like a "relearning" than a *new* learning, because with the New Age it is as if the basis for these had become genetic.

Other books by Raymond Buckland

Anatomy of the Occult
Buckland's Complete Book of Witchcraft
Buckland's Gypsy Fortunetelling Deck
The Tree: Complete Book of Witchcraft
Doors to Other Worlds
Here Is the Occult
The Magick of Chant-O-Matics
A Pocket Guide to the Supernatural
Practical Candleburning Rituals
Practical Color Magick
Scottish Witchcraft
Secrets of Gypsy Dream Reading
Secrets of Gypsy Fortunetelling
Witchcraft Ancient and Modern
Witchcraft from the Inside
Witchcraft . . . the Religion

with Hereward Carrington
Amazing Secrets of the Psychic World
with Kathleen Binger
The book of African Divination
under the pseudonym "Tony Earll"
Mu Revealed

Video
Witchcraft Yesterday and Today

Forthcoming
Gypsy Shamanism
Ray Buckland's Magick Cauldron

For my wife Tara, who has her own
love magick;

and for my mother, who has put up with
all of us wild Romanis.

CONTENTS

Gypsy Potions, Talismans, Amulets and Charms

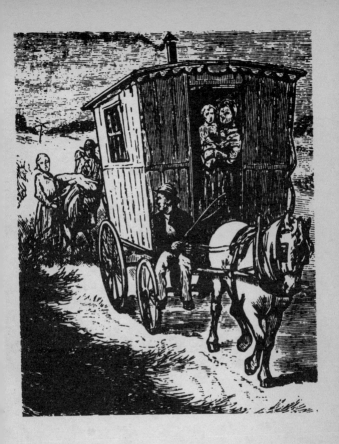

Love is of very great importance to the Gypsies, who are fundamentally complete romantics. And if love somewhat defies tradition, it is the oversight most easily forgiven.

—John-Paul Clébert
The Gypsies

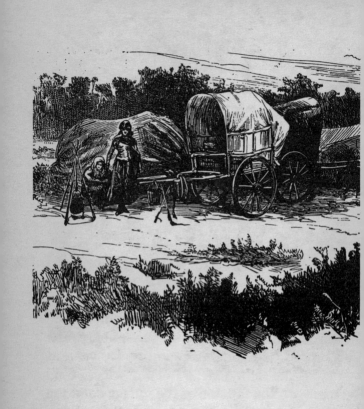

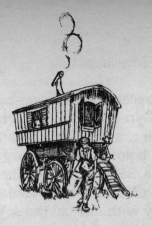

A Magickal Bag of Tricks

More than a dozen pairs of eyes peered from behind curtained windows, watching the line of colorful Gypsy waggons, or *vardos*, pass through the village on their way to the village green. Word spread quickly. The Gypsies had come to town! Every year, at about the same time, a Romani tribe would camp on the far side of the village common land and settle in for a stay of two or three months. While there they would provide the villagers with baskets and clothespins, mend pots and pans, minister to sick animals, and do any odd jobs that needed to be done. But one of the most looked-for services, sought by more villagers than would care admit it,

3

was fortunetelling and the working of magick.

The Gypsies had scarcely had time to set up their camp and light their fires before the more bold of the villagers descended upon them, seeking advice. The women of the tribe were most often consulted, the men being busy with manual tasks. Wives, husbands, lovers, would sit down beside the fire with a Romani *shuvani*, or wise woman, and quickly fall into deep and intense conversation. Occasionally a man or a woman would be invited up the wooden steps into the vardo itself, to watch in awe as the shuvani bent her head over a crystal ball or spread well-worn cards across a table.

The above scene was common in England up until the start of the Second World War. It is not altogether unknown even today. Today's Gypsies are regarded in much the same way as were the Witches of old. This is not a book on Witchcraft, yet there are some similarities between Witches and Gypsies. Today's Witches are struggling mainly to reestablish themselves with regard to their religious beliefs. The original Witches—the *Wicca* and *Wicce* of pre-Christian days (Medieval English *wicche*)—were generally regarded not only as the priesthood but also as the general Wise Ones of the community. In addition to being the local religious leaders, they were also the "doctors" and "lawyers," the healers and advisers. So in the same way that people went to consult with Witches in the past, today they will go to Gypsies for that help and advice—to learn of their future or to obtain help in bringing about something they desire.

For centuries the Gypsies—or the *Romani*, to give them their true name—have traveled the world collecting and dispensing occult knowledge. I have addressed their use of various methods of divination in a previous book (*Secrets of Gypsy Fortunetelling*, Llewellyn Publications, 1988), so in this present volume I would like to present their methods of working magick, specifically love magick.

Magick is simply causing something to happen that you want to happen. As Aleister Crowley put it: "The art or science of causing change to occur in conformity with will." Can this really be done? Very definitely, yes.

There are probably hundreds of ways of working magick, of making things happen. Some methods involve extremely complex and frequently very expensive tools and supplies, together with a need for intimate knowledge of highly esoteric arts, in order to perform them. But there are many other ways (which can be equally effective) that are much more simple, using ordinary everyday materials. These are the ways of the Gypsies. Traveling the roads in their colorful vardos, it would have been difficult, if not impossible, for the Rom to perform exotic ceremonies using the elaborate paraphernalia of ceremonial magick, for example. No, they were far more likely to gather herbs from the hedgerows, fashion crude poppets from bits of rag, or utilize common candles and other household items for their magickal workings.

I have spent some years researching my Romani ancestry. In my explorations up and down England I have encountered a wide variety of magickal beliefs and practices among the Rom. Together with these, I remember things my grandparents did; things that I accepted as part and parcel of growing up yet which now, on reflection, I realize would be out of the ordinary—to say the least—to *gaujos* (non-Gypsies).

● ● ●

Most love magick can be divided into one of three categories:

(1) That which is used during the courting process (e.g., how to get a man or a woman interested in you)

(2) That used after marriage (e.g., how to keep a spouse faithful)

(3) That which applies to family love as a whole (e.g., how to bring harmony between mother and daughter)

I have called these, respectively, The Thrill of the Chase, The Golden Rings, and The Family Circle. By far the largest number of spells and charms fall under the first heading.

One point that needs to be emphasized— especially, perhaps, with regard to The Thrill of the Chase—is the fact that you must *never* try to interfere with another's free will. I will be mentioning this again in the book. We are all individuals, each with our own lives to lead. During your lifetime there may well be times when you feel especially attracted to a particular person and feel strongly tempted to work magick to gain that person's love. If you go ahead and perform that magick, then what you are doing is akin to rape! Working magick is making things happen . . . *making* things happen. To make someone fall in love with you, then, is to force them to fall in love with you, to go *against* their free will. How would you feel if you knew you had been forced to love someone you didn't naturally care for?

So what can you do if you feel strongly about a particular person? The answer is to work on yourself, magickally or however, to make yourself so attractive that the person (or perhaps someone else, someone even better that you hadn't realized was around) will fall for you naturally.

● ● ●

The Gypsies are a fascinating people. I call them The Keepers of the Ancient Mysteries, since they were responsible for the spread of so much occult knowledge over so many centuries. And even now, in today's highly technical civilization, they have a place preserving and dispensing that work. What follows is a little of their knowledge in the realm of love.

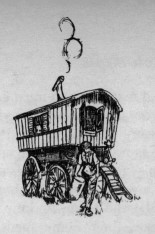

Preparation for Magick

Ingredients

The Gypsies say that the power of magick lies in four simple ingredients. The first of these is the desire/need of the practitioner. The stronger your desire for something to happen and the stronger your need for a thing, then the stronger is the power that you generate towards that goal. We can say, then, that the first ingredient (indeed, the first necessity) for successful magick is *will*.

Along with the will for something to happen must go a certain amount of *concentration*, the second ingredient. It is no good doing anything, least of all magick, in a halfhearted manner. You must concentrate on what you are doing so that you can put that necessary will power into it.

There is no magick wand as described in children's fairy tales. There is no way you can wave a wand or utter a chant or spell, and FLASH! the thing is done. No; even magick takes time. Some spells *can* have effect within 24 hours, but most take longer. Some can take weeks, months, or even more. So the third ingredient is *patience*. Do the work with the necessary will power, give it the required concentration; then be content to sit back and wait for it to have effect . . . and it will take effect.

The final ingredient is simply *secrecy*. Gypsies don't announce when they are doing magick, nor what exactly they are doing. They do it quietly, within the privacy of their vardos. So you, too, should keep secret what you are doing. By running around telling—perhaps bragging to—your friends, you are only weakening the power of what you have done.

In the fields and woods

As you might expect with Gypsy magick, many of these spells are to be done in the

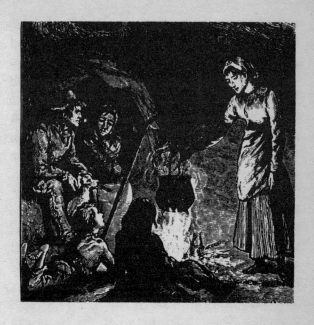

outdoors—out in the fields and the woods, with nature. Some of them call for the use of certain trees or plants. I am well aware that many, if not most, people live in the cities. But don't use this as an excuse for not being able to do a particular spell. If you have a real desire for something to happen (and, as I've said above, you must have that desire, that will, as one of the necessary ingredients), then you will find a way to get to where you have to be or to obtain what you need. Drive out of town if you have to. Or take a bus, taxi, or walk to your closest neighborhood park if that is what is called for. All cities have parks. It's not impossible to get to one. If you find you are making excuses for not being able to follow the directions, then you need to examine your own inner feelings about what you claim you want to make happen.

Any other necessary ingredients are given in the spells themselves as they are described. Heed what is said. Follow the instructions carefully. If you do all this, there is no reason why you shouldn't be as successful as the Gypsies themselves.

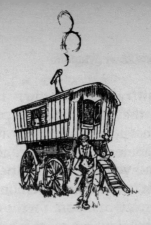

The Thrill of the Chase

In the past it used to be that Gypsy child marriages were arranged. This is seldom the case today, though it does happen on rare occasions. Jean-Paul Clébert speaks of it in *The Gypsies* (Penguin Books, 1967):

Among some Gypsy groups traces remain of the marriage of children before puberty: in general, between eight to fourteen years of age. Such unions are decided upon by the parents and, for a certainty, without the consent of the interested parties. The ceremony is limited to a simple formality, and the children

13

remain with their own families until they have reached puberty. There is never any cohabitation. At the moment of puberty (and when no unavoidable difficulties have arisen), a second ceremony seals the effective union. Yet the custom of precocious marriage is becoming increasingly rare, at least among western Gypsies.

Clébert also speaks of there being three main forms of marriage: viz. "abduction (by force or consent); purchase; mutual consent." The abduction and (outright) purchase forms are little seen today. More generally the parents of a teenage boy will decide which girl in the tribe is most eligible for him (though today the young couple's feelings for one another are given definite consideration). They will then meet with the girl's parents and, should they be favorable, come to an agreement regarding her dowry. From there the couple are regarded as engaged.

There is no engagement ring, as in *gorgio* society, but the girl is given a gold coin that she wears around her neck. This is usually an English sovereign (a Queen Victoria Jubilee sovereign is especially esteemed). The girl could be as young as thirteen, but sixteen is more usual. The boy could be anywhere from sixteen to eighteen.

FOR LOVE

There is someone in whom you are very much interested. He or she seems to notice you but makes no move to develop a relationship. This is not a spell to draw that loved one to you, but more to "open the way," so that if there *is* interest there, he or she will feel free to make advances.

The Seeker should set a wineglass on the table. Then suspend a ring (traditionally the mother's wedding band) from a length of red silk ribbon. Holding the ribbon between thumb and forefinger, as a pendulum, with the elbow resting on the table, let the ring hang in the mouth of the wineglass. Initially you should try to keep the ring still.

In a loud, clear voice, call out your own name followed by the name of your would-be love. Repeat the name of your love twice more (three times in all). Then, thinking of him/her, allow the ring to swing until it "chinks" against the side of the wineglass once for each letter as you spell out the name.

Now take the ribbon and tie it about your neck, allowing the ring to hang down on your chest over the heart. Wear it for three weeks. Every Friday repeat the above ritual. By the end of the third week, if it is meant to be, then the loved one will come to you.

TO DISCOVER YOUR FUTURE SPOUSE

There are one or two (perhaps even three, or more?) people in whom you are interested and who could turn out to be your future spouse. But which one will it be? Here's a way to find out. This ritual should be performed on a night of the Full Moon.

Sit alone in a room that is absolutely quiet. There should be no sound of traffic, television, radio, or anything. On a table in front of you, lay out a piece of black cloth. On the cloth, stand a clear glass tumbler filled with water. The water should be right up to the brim of the glass. To the left of the glass of water have a lighted white candle, which should be the only light in the room.

To the right of it, burn some incense—sandalwood, frankincense, or jasmine are best.

Close your eyes and take two or three really deep breaths. In your mind, see the faces of the possible spouses in front of you, but keep your eyes closed. Say the following, three times:

> *Scry, scry, scry for me.*
> *Bring the face that I must see.*
> *Let me gaze on my future mate*
> *To know which lover will be my*
>   *fate.*

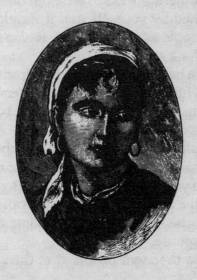

Then, try to clear your mind of everything so that when you open your eyes and gaze down into the water you will be able to accept anything that appears there. And as you do just that, open your eyes and gaze down into the water—you will see the face of the one who is to become your spouse.

THE NAME GAME

To steal apples off a tree is to go "scrumping." For this spell you need to scrump an apple. It therefore has to be taken from a tree not owned by yourself, and it should be as red an apple as you can find. It also should have a long stem on it.

Safe back home again, sit in front of the fire and hold the apple up by its stem. Get a tight grip with one hand and start twisting the apple around with the other. As you twist, call out the letters of the alphabet. You should go fairly quickly, though not too rapidly, because you want to note the letter you call out as the stem parts from the apple. That letter is the initial of the first name of your future spouse.

Toss the stem on the fire, then take a

sharp knife (*choori*) and start to peel the apple. Peel carefully, for you need to get the peel off all in one piece. If it breaks, you must go back and scrump another apple and start all over again.

When the apple is peeled, take the peel in your left hand and toss it over your shoulder so that it lands on the ground behind you. When you turn around to examine it, you will find it has landed in the form of a letter (you may have to study it to make out the letter; it is not always crystal clear). This is the initial of your future spouse's last name.

If the apple peel should break when it lands, then it is going to be a stormy courtship with more than one moment of wanting to call off the whole thing.

THE LOVE PENDULUM

The pendulum can be used for many things: finding lost objects, discovering hidden treasures, divining water, communicating with spirits of the dead, diagnosing illness and prescribing medicine . . . all these and more (see my book *Practical Color Magick*, Llewellyn, 1983). Gypsies use the pendulum quite a lot. One of the uses to which they put it is in determining whether or not a particular lover is the right one for you.

The pendulum itself should be a ring suspended on a length of red silk thread or ribbon. Many girls use their mother's wedding band for the ring (see For Love). The only other thing you need is a connection with the one you are wondering about. This can be an article of his or her clothing, a handkerchief, a watch, ring, or other piece of jewelry, a photograph, or anything similar that has a direct link with the person.

Simply sit with the object, photograph, or whatever in front of you and hold the pendulum over it. It doesn't matter whether or not your elbow rests on the table, but hold the thread so that the ring is suspended about an inch or so above the object. Allow seven inches of the thread between your fingers and the ring.

Concentrate your thoughts on the person you are wondering about. Is he/she the right one for you? Think of all their good qualities, and their bad. Then say:

Av, mi Romani mal,
Pawdel dur chumbas.
Av kitané mansa?

This little verse in *Romanes* (the Gypsy language) can be roughly translated as "Come, my Gypsy friend, over the hills so far away. Will you come along with me?" Repeat it, saying it three times in all.

As you say the verse the pendulum will start to swing. If it swings backwards and forwards, towards you and away from you, then it means "yes," that person is the right one for you. But if it swings from side to side, across you, then it means "no," they are not right for you. With some people the pendulum may swing around in a circle, rather than backwards and forwards. If it does, then clockwise means "Yes" and counterclockwise means "no."

TO ATTRACT A LOVER

This is for when you have a lover but he or she is not as attentive as you would wish. You *know* they love you, but . . .

Sit before a dying fire and gaze into it,

clearing your mind of all but thoughts of your lover. Have a small basket of laurel leaves between your knees. Keeping your gaze fixed on the fire, dip your left hand into the basket, take out a handful of the leaves, and toss them onto the fire. As they burst into flame, chant out loud the following:

Laurel leaves that burn in the fire,
Draw unto me my heart's desire.

Wait till the flames have died down, then repeat the action. Do it a third time. Within 24 hours your lover will come to visit you.

TO RID YOURSELF OF AN UNWANTED LOVER

Some people are wooed by persistent would-be lovers, those who won't take no for an answer and who won't leave them alone. This is the ideal spell for such a situation. It should be done during the waning cycle of the Moon—that is, after the Full Moon and before the New Moon.

Have a roaring fire going, then go outside and pick up two handfuls of dry vervain leaves (you can place them on the ground there ahead of time, if necessary). As you pick them up, shout out the name of the one you wish to be rid of. Turn and go into the house (or cross to the fire if this is all done out in the open) and fling the leaves onto the fire with the words:

Here is my pain;
Take it and soar.
Depart from me now
And offend me no more.

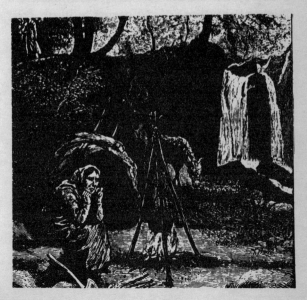

Do this for three nights in a row. You will hear no more from the unwanted one.

TO MAKE YOURSELF KNOWN TO ANOTHER

If you love another and they don't seem to notice, then this can bring you to their attention.

You need to find their footprint in the earth. You then dig up this footprint (more correctly, the earth in which it is impressed). Take the earth to the nearest willow tree and, making a hole in the ground at its base, put the footprint earth into the hole, filling it over with the original dirt. As you are burying the footprint this way, say:

> Many earths on earth there be,
> I make my love known unto thee.
> For he (she) is the flower and I the stem;
> He (I) the cock and me (she) the hen.
> Grow, grow, willow tree!
> Sorrow not for the likes of me.

From then on you will find that the person you yearn for will indeed start to notice you. Where it goes from there, of course, is up to you.

THE REVEALING PEEL

To find if the one you love will become your spouse, do the following. In the morning, as soon as you arise, peel a small lemon. Keep two equal size pieces of the peel, each about the size of a half dollar. Place the pieces with the insides together and the peel sides out, and put them in your right-hand pocket or in your purse. Leave them there all day.

At night, when you undress for bed, take the peel from your pocket or purse and rub the legs of the bed with it. Then place both pieces of peel under your pillow and lay down to sleep. If you dream of your love, then you will surely marry him/her.

The meanings of dreams in general, together with those associated with love, are addressed in my book *Secrets of Gypsy Dream Reading*, which is forthcoming from Llewellyn Publications.

GOOD RIDDANCE!

Here is another good spell for getting rid of an unwanted suitor. Take a small square of paper and write on it the name of the annoying would-be lover. Use black ink for this. Many Gypsies also say that it is best to use one of the old "dip" pens and ink, rather than a modern ballpoint, but you could experiment. Let the ink dry; don't blot it. Then light a white candle and burn the piece of paper in its flame while thinking of the person running away from you. Catch the ashes in something (burning the paper over an ashtray is a good idea) and carry them out to a hillside (you can do this by putting them in a small plastic bag, or similar). There you must place the ashes on the upturned palm of your right hand and hold it up, saying:

> *Winds of the North, East, South,*
> * and West,*
> *Carry these affections to where*
> * they'll be best.*
> *Let her/his heart be open and free,*
> *And let her/his mind be away from*
> * me.*

Then blow on the ashes so that they scatter to the winds.

TO BRING OUT THE
LOVE OF ANOTHER

This is an interesting spell. It does not interfere with another's free will. All it does is give them the courage to state what is on their mind. It is done when you feel very strongly that the person is in love with you but that they hesitate to say so. If it turns out that they are *not* in love with you after all, then it simply won't work, so that's why it doesn't exert undue pressure.

This should be done at the same hour on seven consecutive Fridays, ending on the one closest to the Full Moon (*before* the Moon reaches full, not just after).

Take a pink candle and mark six rings around it, at equal distances apart. This will give you seven sections of candle.

Light the candle and call out the name of the one you think loves you. Then say:

Gana be with me in all that I do.
Gana, please bring me a love who is
*   true.*

> *Give him (her) the strength to put into*
> *words*
> *His (her) feelings, and sing like the song*
> *of the birds.*

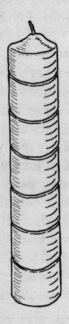

Think about the person for a few moments—think of them coming to you and declaring their love—then repeat the chant. Keep doing this until the candle has burned down to the first line. Then extinguish the candle (by pinching it out, not by blowing) and put it away till next week.

On the final week, keep it up until the candle burns itself out.

RED FOR LOVE

The Gypsies say that to find anything red means luck in love. If you find a piece of red thread, red wool, a red button, or whatever, pick it up and carry it with you for luck. It serves as an amulet.

As you stoop to pick it up, think of the person you love and say:

> *Red is my blood*
> *And red is my heart.*
> *Lucky in love;*
> *Never keep us apart.*

KEY TO THE HEART

It is considered very lucky to find a key. Any sort of key is lucky, but an antique one is especially so. As with the finding of something red, there are words to say at the time of finding it:

*The key to your heart lies on
the ground.
The key to your heart has now
been found.
I lock up your love with the heart
of my own,
I'll guard it forever with the love
I have shown.*

As you say these words, think of the one you love and of the two of you being together forever. Sleep with the key under your pillow for nine nights, carrying it with you during the day. It may then be put in a place of safety.

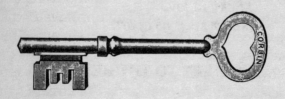

WEDDING DATE

This old custom for finding whether or not you will be married within the coming year is performed on New Year's Eve. The enquirer takes an old shoe and throws it up into the branches of a willow tree. If the shoe falls to the ground again, there will be no wedding within 12 months. But if it catches in the branches and does not fall, then there will be a wedding within the year.

RIVER OF DREAMS

Another way to determine whom you will marry is to use a bowl of water and a flat stick. The bowl should be earthenware and should be filled at least half full of water that has been taken from a flowing stream. A flat stick or piece of wood is then laid across the bowl, from one edge to the other. This represents a bridge over a river or stream.

On the night of a Full Moon, place the bowl of water and stick underneath your bed. Just before you sleep, concentrate your thoughts on an actual footbridge over a stream. Tell yourself that you will dream of it that night. Not only will you dream of the bridge, but you will dream of yourself crossing the bridge and, halfway over, falling off into the water. But have no fear, someone will come and rescue you.

With these expectations, built up in your mind throughout the day and then reinforced just before you sleep, you should have no trouble actually having that dream. The trick then is to remember when you wake who it was who came to your rescue and pulled you from the water. That person is your future spouse.

TO DRAW A LOVER TO YOU

Here again, it's not a case of drawing a specific person to you. Rather, this magick is to draw "someone" to you. No names, though you can certainly specify the *type* of person, e.g., "a dark, six-footer, with a sense of humor and an interest in hang-gliding," or whatever.

The two favorite semiprecious "stones" of the Gypsies are jet and amber. Of course neither one is truly a stone. Jet is an organic product: bituminous coal that can be polished. Amber is the fossilized, hardened resin of the pine tree *Pinus succinifera*, formed during the Eocene period (about 50 million years ago). For this spell you need a piece of amber, and it should (for best results) be a piece with an insect inclusion. If you can't get that, then any piece of amber can be used.

This should be done on a Friday, first thing in the morning when you rise and before you do anything else. Take the piece of amber and hold it in your (closed) left hand. Hold the hand over your heart, close your eyes, and concentrate your thoughts on the type of person you want to attract to you. See him or her in as much detail as you can: height, weight, eye and hair coloring. Think of the interests, sports, activities, you would like them to have. Then see the two of you together, walking hand in hand.

Now kiss the amber and place it in a piece of pink or red silk and wrap it up securely. Carry that with you at all times for the next seven days, sleeping with it under your pillow. Every morning repeat the holding and visualizing, though hold it still wrapped in the silk; don't unwrap it. By the seventh day you will have met someone just like the person you have been wishing for.

TO MAKE YOURSELF AN
OBJECT OF DESIRE

This is a spell that is best performed on May Day, the first of May. As with most of these spells, it can be done by a man or a woman.

Climb to the top of a hawthorn tree and break off about 12 inches of the topmost branch. Carry it back down to the ground with you. With the broken end of the limb, mark a circle on the ground on the east side of the tree. The circle should be about three feet in diameter. Stand in the circle facing east and, holding the twig above your head, say the following:

> *Oprĕ the rooker, adrĕ the vesh*
> *Si chiriklo ta chirikli;*
> *Telĕ the rook adrĕ the vesh*
> *Si piramno ta piramni."*

(Roughly translated this means, "Over the tree and into the woods are male and female birds. Under the tree and into the woods are male and female sweethearts."[1])

---

[1]George Borrows, in his 1874 book *Romano Lavo Lil*, gives a similar rhyme as part of a song called "The Squire and the Lady." He does not give a literal translation but has obviously rather tried to make a poetic rendering into English. He gives it as "I see, I see upon the tree, the little male and female dove; Below the tree, I see, I see, the lover and his lady love."

Now stick the branch into the ground, in the middle of the circle, and walk away without looking back.

TO GIVE A WOULD-BE
LOVER COURAGE

Here is another example of sympathetic magick. This spell is excellent should you have a lover who is extremely shy and very reluctant to declare his or her love.

As in the previous spell (To Make Yourself an Object of Desire) you need a piece of branch from a tree. This time you need not climb to the top of the tree to get it. You should, however, break it off the tree yourself, rather than picking up a twig that has fallen. Actually you are going to need two twigs. They must come from an oak tree and need be only about six inches long for one, and three or four inches for the other. You are going to use these as a base for making a doll figure to represent your lover.

On the larger piece of wood scratch, paint, or write in some fashion the name of your lover. On the shorter piece, scratch the word *HEART*. Now take the smaller twig and lay it across the larger, about two inches from the top, to form a cross. Tie it in place with a hair, or several hairs, from his or her head. Stick the wooden figure into the ground at the foot of the oak tree and lay down a circle of acorns all around it.

Kneel in front of it, facing it and the tree, and say:

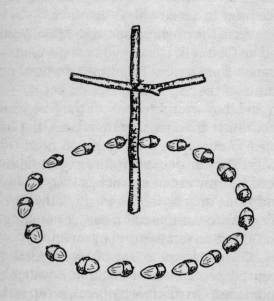

Fill your heart with the strength
that is here;
Feel the oak driving out all fear.
Say the words to bring joy to the
heart,
And never again will we be apart.

Leave then and return the following day. If the stick figure still stands, kneel and repeat the rhyme. Do this for seven days in a row. If the figure stands throughout, then all will be well and you will soon be together. But if for any reason the figure is not standing any time you go to it, then there will be some obstruction to the two of you getting together.

TO MAKE SOMEONE THINK OF YOU

For this you need a small mirror, like a woman's purse makeup mirror. Take a photograph of yourself and put it *behind* the mirror. Then take a photograph of the person you want to think of you and place it face down against the *front* of the mirror (so that the two photographs are facing one another but with the mirror between them). Wrap up the three in a piece of red paper or cloth, and fasten it securely so that it cannot come undone and the photographs cannot come away from the mirror.

Take the package to the home of the person you want to think of you and hide it somewhere in the house, where it will not be discovered. It used to be that it would be hidden in the rafters or in the thatch of the roof, but these days you have to do the best you can.

Some Gypsies say that you don't even have to take it to the person's home. They say that just the fact of having the pictures fastened to the mirror, back and front, will do the trick. However, others say that it is essential that it be placed in the person's home, so if you want to play it safe, I would suggest getting it in there.

TO ENCOURAGE A SHY LOVER

Gypsies say that feeding a shy lover beet-root will give him or her confidence. I have also heard it said that tomatoes will make him/her more amorous. However, a spell that is worked quite frequently for this sort of a situation is as follows.

Obtain the lover's handkerchief, or a small piece of clothing that has been worn next to the skin. Gather at least seven acorns and wrap them in the material, tying it around with a length of red wool. Sleep with this package under your pillow for seven consecutive nights; then on the eighth day, go into the woods and stuff it into a cleft in a tree. This could be a squirrel's hole, a gash caused by lightning, or some form of natural hole in the trunk. If you cannot find such a place, then it is permissible to wedge it firmly into a fork, so long as it is a tight fit. The type of tree is not important, though I suspect that oak would be best.

Now, starting in the east, walk three times around the tree calling out your lover's name repeatedly as you walk. Then walk away without looking back.

TO FAN A SPARK INTO A FLAME

Lay down a circle of stones, each about the size of a potato. The circle should be 21 inches in diameter. In the center of the circle make a fire.

Take a length of wood, about two or

three inches thick and about a foot in length. Carve the name of your lover along its length.

When the fire has been burning well and is starting to settle down, put the piece of wood across the middle of the fire, laying it east-west. Let the wood catch alight and burn, but all the time it is burning look at it and imagine your lover with his or her love growing in intensity for you. Do not poke the fire at all but allow the stick to lay there across the top all the while it is burning. When the wood has burned at least half through, sprinkle some sugar along its length and call out your lover's name. You will find that the sugar causes the wood to flare up again. Repeat this, sprinkling and calling seven times in all. Don't rush it; it will take awhile for the wood to burn all the way through.

When the wood has finally finished burning and there is nothing left but hot ash—and not before—pour clean water over the fire to completely deaden it.

TO NARROW THE FIELD

Three possible lovers . . . which one to choose? Before going to sleep at night, write down the names of the contenders on separate slips of paper and place them under your pillow. When you get into bed, lie with eyes closed and concentrate on each of them, one at a time. Slip a hand under the pillow and pull out one of the slips. Do not look at it (it's best to do this when the light is out, anyway) but drop it on the floor beside the bed.

In the morning, slip your hand under the pillow again and pull out another piece of paper. Drop that on the floor also. The remaining name is the one for you. You can do this with more than three names, of course, pulling out more than one each time, just so long as only one is left at the end.

A variation on the above was mentioned by one Gypsy *rakli* I spoke to in Kent. She said that if a girl writes the names of all her boyfriends on one slip of paper and then goes to sleep with the paper tucked between her breasts, she will dream of the one who will become her husband.

TO BROADEN THE FIELD

It can be a problem when you have too many suitors and you need to narrow the field. But what about when the reverse is true? What do you do when you have just one, or perhaps two, people wanting you but you feel you would like a far larger group from which to choose? How do you broaden the field?

One way is to do as the Gypsies do and work a little magick. From a piece of pink cloth, make a drawstring pouch about three inches by six inches. On one side of the pouch embroider your initials (or full name). On the other side embroider a heart. This embroidery should be done with red silk thread. Place a large acorn in the pouch together with two smaller ones (or however many admirers you presently have).

Every morning when you rise, go out into the woods and pick up the first acorn you find. Place it in the pouch with the others. Do this until you have a total of eight acorns— one to represent yourself and seven others to represent seven admirers. Do this gathering as soon as you get out of bed, before you have coffee or anything to eat.

Every night, from the start, sleep with the bag under your pillow. During the day wear it suspended from a red ribbon so that it hangs down under your clothing against your skin. (Some say it should be hanging over your heart, others say it should be down between your legs.)

Within three days of completing the collection of acorns you will start obtaining new admirers. You can eventually have as many as seven. If you decide you want to stop at six, or five, or fewer, just stop wearing the bag. You can then get to know them all and make your choice!

But what do you do if you live in the city, and there are no oak trees close by? First of all, make quite sure that there really are no oak trees. It's surprising how many cities do have parks within easy reach that we just don't notice or simply assume are not there. But if you really don't have access to an area where you might find acorns, then simply work with something else. I have known city dwellers who used such diverse items as coins (it's incredible how many pennies get dropped and left lying), soft-drink bottle caps, pebbles, or nuts and bolts. There was one young lady I knew who picked up discarded styrofoam coffee cups and cut out the bottoms of them. Washing them, she had styrofoam discs instead of acorns in her pouch. The first one (a new one) she had written her name on.

Look around. See what's out there. As with so much of magick, it's really the thought/feeling and the action that you put into it that generates the force for the magick, so whether it's acorns or pop-tops, you should have success.

TO CARRY YOUR LOVER TO YOU ACROSS LAND AND SEA

There is nothing worse than being separated from the one you love. It often happens that the Rom get separated. When they do, they work a little magick to speed their reunion.

Take a half walnut shell and drill a small hole near the edge (see illustration). Thread a length of red thread through the hole and tie a knot in the end so that it won't come back out. Fill a bucket with water and float the walnut shell. Holding the end of the thread, say:

Come to me, over land and sea.
Return at once to my side.
By Gana's love do I make this plea,
That together we may abide.

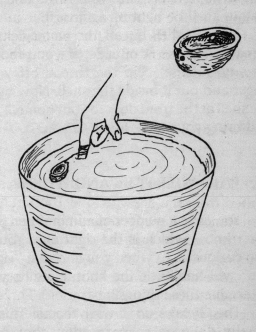

Hold the end of the thread in your hand and put your hand over the pail of water, your index finger pointing down into it. With the shell at the outer edge, start to stir the water so that as you stir, the thread winds onto your extended finger.

Repeat the rhyme, saying it three times

in all, by which time the thread should have wound completely onto your finger and the walnut shell be tight up against it.

Lift the shell out of the water by the thread and take it outside (if you are not already outside). Slip the thread off your finger and put it inside the shell. Now bury the shell at the front door to your home. This will bring your lover home to you.

WHO WILL IT BE AND WHEN?

You have a number of admirers and just don't know which is the right one. You're also curious as to when you and that "right one" will finally tie the knot. How do you determine these things?

The Gypsies do it with acorns. This is usually done on a Wednesday, though a Friday would also be good. First, gather as many acorns as you have admirers, plus one to represent yourself. Then take a sharp knife and scratch the initial of each person, one on each acorn.

Fill a bowl with water. Take up the acorns and, holding them in your hands, concentrate on the people they represent. See each of them in turn and study the things about them that attract you. Now open your hands and drop the acorns, all together, into the bowl of water. The acorn that floats closest to yours is the person most right for you.

Next remove all the acorns from the bowl and throw out all but yours and the "finalist." Hold these two in your cupped hands, over your heart, and say:

Gana, Gana, when will it be?

Then throw the two of them back into the bowl. If they stay floating close together (within about three inches of one another), then you will be marrying within the year. But if they float a good distance apart, then it will be a long engagement.

PEAS IN A POD

Young Gypsy girls, when preparing vegetables for cooking, will look especially carefully at the peas they are shelling. If you should find seven peas in a pod, then keep that pod.

Place one half of the pod over the door

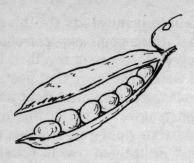

of your vardo—or the main door into your house. Keep the other half pod in your pocket, or somewhere on your person.

The first eligible male to enter your home will be drawn immediately to you, and will be the one you will eventually marry.

CARDS AND LOVE

Playing cards and Romani tarot decks are used a great deal by the Gypsies (see *Secrets of Gypsy Fortunetelling* and *The Buckland Gypsy Fortunetelling Deck*). They are especially used for divining what may lie ahead in the way of love for a young man or woman. I give many layouts in the above-mentioned books. There is one additional layout, how-

ever, that is used by a few shuvanis when a
person is in doubt about which of two suitors
is the right one.

The Right Choice

One card is chosen for the Significator.
This is one of the court cards: for an older
man, one of the Kings; for an older woman,
one of the Queens; for a young man or woman, one of the Jacks. The actual suit is determined by the person's coloring: white skin =
Diamonds, medium fair skin = Hearts, medium dark skin = Clubs, dark skin = Spades.

The Significator is removed and the rest
of the cards are shuffled by the person seeking
advice. After shuffling, the cards are cut with
the left hand, to the left, into two piles. The
Reader picks them up in reverse order and deals
out the top three cards to the left of the Significator; the next three to its right; next three
below the first set, on the left; next three on
the right; and so on till three sets of three are
on each side of the Significator (see illustration on p. 50). Cards should be face up.

The cards on the *left* represent the younger
of the two suitors; those on the *right* the
older. The first thing the Reader does is to

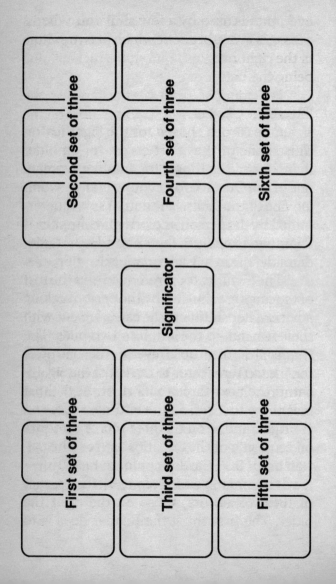

add up the total values of each set of cards. This will give a preliminary idea of the value of the person to the inquirer, the higher value being the better one.

For example: Let's say the cards on the left are 6, 9, 7; 4, A, J; 2, 3, K and those on the right are 10, 2, Q; 4, 6, 7; K, A, 9. Those on the left add up $6 + 9 + 7 + 4 + 1 + 11 + 2 + 3 + 13 = 56$. Those on the right: $10 + 2 + 12 + 4 + 6 + 7 + 13 + 1 + 9 = 64$. Obviously the one on the right is higher.

Now look at the cards themselves. If there is a preponderance of court cards on one side, then that is very much in that person's favor. It shows they will be a person of consequence, with much authority. Yet Aces mean major achievements, single special achievements, so these must also be weighed. If red cards outnumber black, then the person's heart rules more than their head (black outnumbering red, the reverse). For individual meanings to cards, please see my above-mentioned books; but from what I have just said, a good general evaluation can be gathered. Often this is sufficient to show the Inquirer that one suitor is far and away a better match than the other.

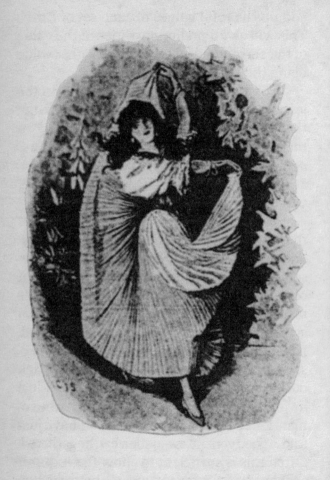

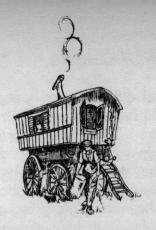

The Golden Rings

It wasn't uncommon for two Romani families to make a marriage arrangement, and agree on a dowry, only to find that the young couple concerned did not care for one another at all. Or worse, that they were in love with someone else. Many times the solution for the son or daughter concerned was to elope with their true love. When this happened the couple would stay away for several weeks but eventually return to seek forgiveness. Invariably they would be severely reprimanded in front of the whole tribe, but then accepted back as husband and wife. If the son or daughter had done the unforgivable of eloping with a *gauji* or *gaujo*, then they would seldom, if ever, be accepted back and would have to travel the roads alone from then on. This was more often the case when a Gypsy girl married outside the blood than if a boy did so. If a non-Gypsy woman (gauji) was accepted into the tribe, she would have to show complete submission to her mother-in-law and was generally forbidden to leave the camp for any reason whatsoever.

But if all had gone according to plan, the dowry was paid and then festivities began, with Gypsies traveling from miles away to attend the wedding (it is amazing how quickly the Rom can get messages out to far-flung members of the tribe when necessary). Rather than a Best Man and Maid of Honor, a married couple is chosen to act as sponsors. They are somewhat like the godparents at a baptism in that they will be available to help, advise and give support to the couple from then on.

The actual ceremony varies tremendously from tribe to tribe. The central point occurs when the two young people promise always to remain true to one another. In fact, in some tribes that is really all there is to the ceremony! In others there are featured exchanges of bread and/or salt, red *diklos* (headscarves) and red flowers. There are records of couples cutting their wrists and mingling their blood, tying their arms together with a red cloth, but this is very rare today.

Shortly after birth a Romani boy is given two golden earrings, which he always wears. At the wedding ceremony he gives his bride the right earring. It is therefore possible to tell if a Rom is married or not by whether he wears one or two earrings.

In some Gypsy weddings the couple will jump over a besom, or broomstick. In others it is long branches of broom they leap across. This obviously ties in with magickal beliefs, since broom figures in many charms for fertility and for protection from evil spirits. Also magickal is the eating of a cake, or small loaf, by the bride and groom, into which has been baked some of their blood.

There is usually no wedding ring (or rings) given. The bride's finger is entwined with a small posy or ring of flowers. At a later date this will be replaced with a gold ring when the two of them, together, have earned the money to pay for it, showing their partnership in life.

The celebrations may go on for days, with much feasting, dancing and singing.

This is a time for general truce, with all disagreements and quarrels forgotten. Songs and dances play an important part in the celebration. In his book *Gypsy Demons and Divinities* (Citadel Press, NJ 1973) Elwood Trigg says:

> Special words, gestures, songs and dances called *debla, alborea, cachucha* and *mosca* form the most important part of a very ancient magical rite. The debla contains remnants of various incantations, probably brought by the Gypsies from India for the purpose of appealing for the blessing of the beneficent spirit or spirits who are thought to preside over all such ceremonies. The alborea is likewise very primitive and may very well be the predecessor of flamenco. The other two parts of the rite, though less magical in their purpose, still contain elements considered necessary to the completion of the total ceremony.

The bride's virginity is of paramount importance. At many Romani weddings the bride and groom retire early on in the celebrations, with the groom returning some time later displaying the bedsheet (or more frequently, a white silk handkerchief) with the telltale bloodstain. This is then cause for even greater rejoicing!

TO SEAL THE KNOT

To keep the marriage solid, with both partners forever faithful to one another, perform this ritual which, interestingly, is almost identical to an ancient Witchcraft cord magick spell (see *Buckland's Complete Book of Witchcraft*, page 162).

The spell is done with a three-foot length of red ribbon. The wife ties the first knot, the husband the second, the wife the third, and so on.

Tying the first knot in the middle of the ribbon, both partners say, "With this first knot we start our marriage."

—————————X—————————

Tying the second knot at one end, they both say, "With this second knot we pledge our love."

X_____X_____

The third knot is tied at the other end. They both say, "With this third knot we promise to be forever true."

X_____X_____X

The four knot is tied between the middle and one end, with the words, "With this fourth knot we entwine our hearts."

X_____X_____X_____X

Tying between the center and the other end, they say, "With this fifth knot we cling together."

X_____X_____X_____X_____X

The sixth is tied between one of the end knots and the one next to it, saying, "With this sixth knot we support one another."

X__X__X_____X_____X_____X

At the other end, between the end and

the knot next to it, "With this seventh knot we join our souls."

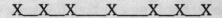

Between the center and the one next to it, "With this eighth knot we protect one another from all ills."

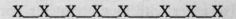

And with a final knot between the center and the other quarter one, "With this ninth knot we become as one."

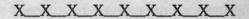

The knotted ribbon is then put away in a safe place.

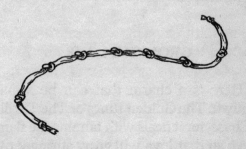

TYING A LOVE KNOT

There is another magickal working that is done by knotting a ribbon. It is somewhat different from the above, however, as you will see. This spell is to ensure that your (male) lover remains faithful only to you.
Take a length of red silk ribbon *the same length as his erect penis.* How you determine this (whether with or without his knowledge) is up to you. Place the ribbon under your pillow so that it is there while you make love. Then, when he is asleep, take out the ribbon and tie seven knots in it. Presumably this represents one for each day of the week, though the number seven has special significance for the Gypsies, occurring in a number of places. So long as you keep the ribbon safe, with the knots intact, he will remain faithful to you.

GROWING LOVE

Here is a charm that can be applied equally to The Golden Rings or The Thrill of the Chase, for it deals with fanning the flames of love so that love will grow stronger over the months and years and blossom into something truly beautiful.

Take a flower bulb. The type is left up to you. Gypsies prefer tulip, hyacinth, or crocus (though the crocus is more correctly a corm, rather than a bulb). Plant the bulb either in the ground or in a pot. If it is in a pot, then it should be a pot that has not been previously used. As you plant the bulb, speak the name of your love seven times. Lay the bulb gently in the earth and cover it, looking upon it as though you were tucking your loved one into a bed.

Over the length of time it takes for the bulb to develop, grow and flower, take good care of it. Every day stand over it and say "I give my heart to my love" three times, and call out his or her name seven times. As the flower grows, so will the love grow, until it eventually blossoms out in all its glory.

MARRIAGE FOUNDATION

Man's best friend may be thought to be the dog, but the Romani's best friend is his horse. The horse is prized above many things. Indeed, a vardo—and therefore the Gypsy family—can go nowhere without one. Tied in with this, as you'll see, is the fact that the Gypsies have a great reverence for the Moon. Diana—known in some areas as Gana—was honored by generations of Gypsies. She is always associated with the Moon.

The common equation between the horse and the Moon is the horseshoe. It is moon-shaped and, perhaps because of this, is believed to bring many blessings from the Moon Goddess. We are all familiar with the idea of hanging a horseshoe over the door to bring good luck. Well, to the Rom this is far more than just a superstition. It really does work.

At gaujo weddings a silver cardboard horseshoe frequently is featured. Silver, of course, is the metal associated with the Moon, so again we have the tie-in with the Goddess. At many Gypsy weddings the couple is presented with a small (pony's) polished silver horseshoe. This becomes one of their prize possessions. It is kept and guarded, for to lose it would bode ill for the marriage.

If you hang a horseshoe over your door, be sure to hang it with the points upward. This is to keep in the "luck" ("blessings" is a better word). If you hang it with the points downward, the luck will all run out.

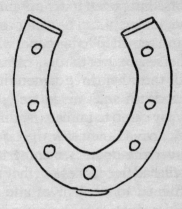

Many Gypsy women have a small silver or gold horseshoe charm on a bracelet or necklace. It is a very popular talisman among the Rom.

In his book *Gypsy Demons and Divinities*, Elwood Trigg relates a story told by German Gypsies. They say that there existed four evil demons known as Unhappiness, Bad Luck, Bad Health, and Death. The horseshoe became a good-luck charm because of a Gypsy Chief's encounter with them. One day, when out riding, this young Chief was set upon and chased by the demon Bad Luck. As they galloped along, one of the shoes from the

Chief's horse happened to fly off and strike the demon, killing him. The Chief retrieved the shoe and returned to his tribe, where he hung the horseshoe over the door of his vardo. Meanwhile the other three demons heard of Bad Luck's death and immediately headed for the Gypsy camp to punish the Chief. But when they arrived they saw the horseshoe hanging over the door. Remembering that the horse still had three shoes left, they became very frightened for their lives and turned and ran. Ever since then the horseshoe has been regarded as a very powerful protective charm against all forms of evil.

TO KEEP A SPOUSE FAITHFUL

If you have suspicions about your wife's or husband's faithfulness, then work this old Romani spell. It is said to never fail.

Take two large potatoes and scrub them clean. Cut them in half lengthwise. You will be using just one half from each potato, so you can throw away or cook the other two halves.

With a sharp-pointed knife, scratch your own name on one half. On the other half scratch your spouse's name. Place the two halves (cut) face to face so that it resembles one whole potato. Stick a new three-inch nail through the potato, with the head of the nail on the spouse's side and the point coming through on your side. Then bind the whole thing around with red silk thread.

In the light of the Moon (it doesn't have to

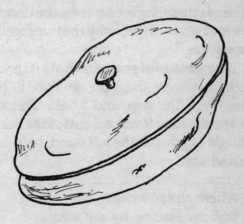

be full, but it should be waxing, i.e., moving from new to full), go out into the garden or to some piece of common land and bury the potato at least seven inches deep.

So long as the potato remains undisturbed, so will your marriage.

TO DRAW AND KEEP
TWO PEOPLE CLOSE

Another charm to keep a married couple together, drawing them ever closer to one another, is this simple one. It can be done by either husband or wife, or by the two together if they wish.

Take a blade of grass and hold it in your mouth, between the lips, so that it protrudes. Face the east and kneel. Think of your spouse for a few moments; then taking the blade of grass in the left hand, hold it up high and say:

Where the sun rises
Will my love be by my side.

Replace the grass in the mouth. Turn to the west and again kneel. Again think of your spouse for a few moments then, taking the grass in the right hand, hold it up high and say:

Where the sun goes down
Will we ever be together.

Again replace the grass blade in the mouth and stand. Face north and think of the two of you together. Then remove the blade once again. The blade should now be cut into fine pieces and mixed in with some food, which is eaten by both husband and wife.

TO HEAL A RIFT

This spell is somewhat similar to the one, To Keep a Spouse Faithful, but uses an apple rather than potatoes.

If you and your spouse have had a tiff, or even a major argument, obtain a large red apple and cut it in half. The cut should not be lengthwise (from stem to tip) but *across* the apple. Now take two cloves—one to represent yourself and the other to represent your spouse. Hold them, one in each hand, for a few moments and concentrate on your true love for one another. Then stick the cloves into the cut surfaces of the apple—one in each half. Put the two halves of the apple back together again and push a thin stick (preferably myrtle or hazel) through the core to hold it together.

Now take the apple down to the banks of a river, stream or lake and throw it out into the middle with the words:

> Gana, rejoin us,
> Even as the apple has been
>   rejoined.
> Bring us the sweetness of Love
> And of Life.
> And let all disharmony
> Be washed away forever.

TO FORGIVE A MISTAKE

Most of us make mistakes at one time or another. Sometimes between two lovers it is not easy to forgive, depending upon the enormity of the mistake. This little ritual will make it easier and, in so doing, will bring you both together again, even closer than before. The working of this magick requires the action of both parties, showing the forgiveness of the one and the remorse of the other.

Take three candles—two white and one

red. Light the candles, then sit facing one another holding hands (left hand in left, right hand in right). Let the guilty party admit his or her guilt, and let the injured party say "I love you. I forgive you." Then release hands and place a coin (Gypsies use a silver coin) in a dish. The guilty party takes a white candle and allows wax to fall from it onto the coin. The injured party does the same with the other white candle. Then the guilty party takes up the red candle and allows its wax to fall on the gathered white wax on the coin, saying:

> *Let my love for you cover the hurt I*
> *have caused, that evermore we may*
> *be as one.*

Take hands again and kiss over the coin. The coin should then be taken out and buried in the ground at the foot of a willow tree.

For this ritual you can use small candles; in fact, even birthday-cake candles will do the job.

TO BECOME CLOSE FRIENDS

One of the joys of my own life is the fact that not only are my wife and I married and in love, but we are also each other's best friend. This is not as common in marriage as one might think. Indeed, many husbands and wives are almost strangers to one another. The Rom have a way of bringing this close friendship between husband and wife. They call it *kitanépen*.

The Romani headscarf is called a *diklo*. Both women and men wear it—the women on their head and the men either around their head or around the neck. For this spell both husband and wife must be wearing a diklo on their head as they make love. After the lovemaking, the two diklos are used to wipe their genitals and are then laid one on top of the other and rolled up. They are then knotted at either end so that they cannot unroll.

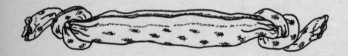

The knotted diklos must now be kept in a safe place—most Rom wives keep them in the bottom of their linen drawer. Once a year (I would suggest on your wedding anniversary) they are taken out, *but not unknotted*, and placed under the bed (i.e., mattress) while the couple make love.

TO BRING A CHILD

Take an egg and carefully make a small hole in each end. Husband and wife kiss, then hold the egg between them, each covering an end with their mouth. The husband now blows into the eggshell and blows the raw egg out of it into the wife's mouth. It will help if she sucks as he blows. She then swallows it (raw egg really isn't too awful). The empty shell is put to one side, and husband and wife make love.

After their lovemaking the couple take out the empty eggshell and bury it in the ground, at least seven inches deep.

TO INCREASE THE NUMBER
OF CHILDREN

Many Gypsies feel that a large family is a happy family, and therefore they like to have lots of children. In order to bring this about, there are a number of magickal workings found in different Romani tribes.

One such rite involves the drinking of a glass of water and brandy mixed with the herb comfrey (*Symphytum officinale*). The water and brandy is mixed half and half. A good pinch of the powdered rootstock of comfrey is sprinkled on it. Both husband and wife must drink from the same glass, the wife drinking first. Immediately after drinking they must make love. This should be repeated three nights in a row to ensure that the wife will not only become pregnant but will continue to conceive on a regular basis.

Another ritual also involves brandy. This time, however, the brandy is sprinkled on the bed linen and in a circle around the bed before the husband and wife make love. Also sprinkled around the bed (but not on the bed linen) is coal dust and French chalk. This, too, should be done on three successive nights. The sprinkling around the bed is done in a clockwise direction.

Another spell to ensure that the home will be filled with children is performed on the birth of the firstborn. The baby is brought into the home and laid down first on the threshold, then on the hearth, and then in each and every corner of every room. When it is laid down, the father must sprinkle crumbs of bread around it and ask the gods for "wealth of life."

Incidentally, if an abortifacient should be necessary at any time, then a tea made either of tansy leaves or of pennyroyal leaves should do the trick.

FOR A WIFE TO RETAIN HER BEAUTY

Romani women are invariably very beautiful, and their menfolk are justly proud of them. The women therefore go out of their way to retain their beauty. They do this using a combination of beauty treatments and magickal spells.

The beauty treatment indulged in by nearly all *juvvels* and young *raklis* (women and young girls) is that of washing the face with early morning dew. For some this is an automatic everyday ritual throughout the month. For others it is a magickal act that is done religiously (literally?) but only through the waxing cycle of the Moon.

The dew is not "gathered" in any way. It is simply a case of the woman kneeling, or even lying, on the ground, wetting her hands with dew and then rubbing it all over her face. I have even seen some girls who lay flat on the grass and rub their faces directly onto the dew.

The second most popular method is using the white of an egg. The egg is separated and its white is beaten in a white china dish. It is then applied to the face and neck and allowed to dry. It remains there for about 15 minutes before it is washed off with pure spring water or water from a running stream. The remaining yolk is taken out and buried at the foot of a rosebush.

In another spell, which is purely magickal, the woman stands naked in the light of the Full Moon and goes through the actions of bathing herself. She should be looking up at the Moon throughout this. If a cloud passes across the Moon, it is a bad sign. If the Moon remains free and clear throughout the rite, she will become more and more lovely every day. As she "bathes," the woman says:

Moon, Moon, beautiful Moon,
Look down on me, smile down
* on me.*
Moon, Moon, grant my boon,
And keep true beauty unto me.

FOR A MAN TO RETAIN HIS VIRILITY

There is an old charm that, I am told, originated in Spain. It is used when a man loses his virility. It must be performed by the man himself, rather than by a shuvani working on his behalf. It is done at the side of a stream, with the man naked.

Dip a large pitcher into the running stream and draw off water, working *with* the current (rather than against it). Then gather three twigs, one each from three different trees, and stand them in the water. Stir the water with the twigs, saying:

Pani, pani, tove mandi wusher;
Naflipen shav ta muk mandi sasti.
(literally, "Water, water, wash me
* clean;*

Illness run away and leave me
    healthy.")

Take the three twigs and throw them
into the stream. Then wash all over with the
water and pour what remains back into the
stream.

TO BRING LOVE INTO AN
ARRANGED MARRIAGE

It used to be that many Romani marriages
were arranged, when the prospective bride
and bridegroom were still children, between
the parents of the boy and the girl. If this
happened, then the shuvani was frequently
called upon to bring love to the couple so
that they might be happy with one another.
Here is one way that this was done.

The shuvani would take an undergar-
ment from each of them, preferably soaked in
sweat. These she would place together and wrap
in a clean white cloth. At the side of a stream,
she would dig a hole and lay the package in
the bottom of it. On top of the cloth she
would place a white egg, a red rose, and an
acorn. She would then fill in the hole.

Every Full Moon for three months the shuvani would dance on top of the buried articles. The dance, apparently extemporaneous, would be preceded and followed by a short period of meditation, presumably on the growing love of the couple.

TO DRAW HUSBAND AND WIFE CLOSER TOGETHER

The idea of working magick on a footprint is found universally and, among the Romani people, is not limited to "the thrill of the chase" (see To Make Yourself Known). It is also used by them for drawing husband and wife closer together.

Find a good, well-defined footprint left by your spouse and carefully dig up the earth containing it. Place the earth in a flowerpot, adding more earth if necessary. In the pot, plant a marigold. This you must then tend and nurture. As the marigold matures and blossoms, so will the marriage.

This particular magick was found among Gypsies in the southwest of England. The same spell is found with the Gypsies of Yorkshire (northern England), except that there they say you should also make a fine foot-print of your own and then mix that with the one left by your spouse.

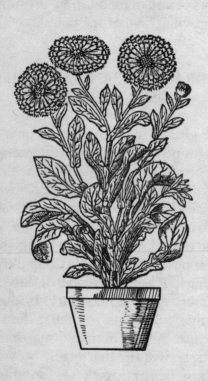

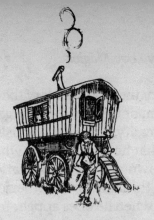

The Family Circle

Manfri Frederick Wood, a founding member of the Gypsy Council, and for many years its president, said that he had never met a Gypsy who had a hobby. The reason was that life itself is a hobby to the Rom. They believe in living life to its fullest, and in trying to take an intelligent interest in every job they do, they find there is no need to do anything just to "kill time." As Wood says:

A Gaujo will go out for a walk or a drive merely for the sake of walking or driving—but a Gypsy won't; he must have some reason for doing so; he is studying the lay of the land, or the movements of the game-keeper, or the habits of the game in the locality; or he is advertising the fact that he is in the area, where he is known and has a reputation for doing this, that, or the other job . . . Even when he does appear to be at play—for instance singing and dancing, gambling, or doing a chop—it is with a view to something extra in the pocket.[2]

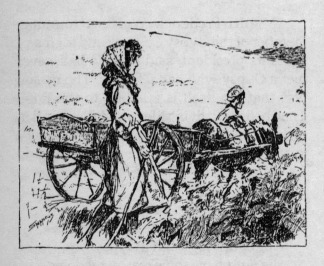

[2]*In the Life of a Romany Gypsy*, Routledge Kegan Paul, London, 1973

The same holds true for the whole family. Even the children seldom play, in the strict sense of the word. They work along with the rest of the family. They may do basketwork, peg-making, artificial flower-making, wood-carving or metalwork; they may work with animals, or do dyeing, hedging, ditching, or perhaps *dukkering* (fortunetelling). The family works as a unit. Boys will help their fathers with the horses and, from a very early age, will learn how to make deals. Girls similarly learn domestic chores from their mothers and also how to tell fortunes and work simple magick. There is a special closeness in a Romani family not found anywhere else.

Yet as with any family, there are times when the closeness is threatened. There are times when magick is needed, and used, to reinforce the family ties. Here are some of the charms and spells used for those times.

HOME HARMONY

Prepare a pot of tea (size depending upon the size of the family, as you will see) made from valerian root herb (*Valeriana officinalis*). The cut and sifted form of the herb is most useful, since it can be easily strained through a regular tea strainer. Dried herbs can be used, but fresh herbs are better. Use about an ounce of herb to a pint of water. The herb should be broken up in a pestle and mortar to release the active principles. Since valerian is one of the deeper essences, you may need to simmer the tea for about an hour, after which time about half the water will have evaporated. Incidentally, do not use an aluminum vessel. Use glass (Pyrex), earthenware, enamel, or stainless steel.

When ready, pour into a teapot and top-up with hot water. Then with everyone sitting in a circle, the mother should pour a cup of tea for each family member; but make sure that at least half the tea is left in the pot (this is where the size of the pot comes in). All drink their tea. Then take what remains in the teapot and sprinkle a little of the tea in every corner of every room in the house: in the corners of the rooms and alcoves, and in the corners of all the larger closets (such as clothes closets and pantries).

When this has been done, all the family members should stand in the kitchen with hands joined, and the mother, or eldest female, should say:

Peace be unto this house
And peace be with all who dwell
  herein.
Let harmony be forever here,
And let love abound.

FAMILY TOGETHERNESS

This little spell can be done for two lovers, for all family members, or for any two or more individuals. Many Gypsies use it when, for example, there is a rift between mother and daughter or an argument between husband and wife.

Cut a lock of hair from the head of each person concerned. This should be cut during the waxing phase of the Moon (growing from new to full). Put the two locks of hair together and tie them with a red silken thread. The thread should be wound around the hair at least seven times before it is tied. Wrap the tied hair in a small square of white silk and then bury it at a crossroads (it doesn't have to be buried right in the center of the crossed roads; alongside the cross is fine).

TO BRING ABOUT A REUNION

Romani families, or tribes, though wandering the country most of the year, would occasionally stop at a particularly favorite campground for two or three months at a time. Frequently this campground was a favorite of other branches of the tribe, and sometimes there was a grand reunion that took place when the different groups came together there. Many Gypsies, especially the older ones, looked forward to these reunions, to again meeting with old friends and to sharing their stories, their adventures, their tales of sorrow and joy. Here is a spell that was sometimes worked to bring about such a gathering, particularly if it had been a hard winter and support, comfort, and advice was needed. This magick is worked by the mother of the family when cooking a meal (usually hedgehog or rabbit stew) during the waxing of the Moon.

All potatoes to be used should be cut lengthwise, rather than crosswise, and thrown into the family cookpot along with a pinch each of allspice, thyme, and mace. Onion can be used but not garlic. Carrots, turnips and similar root crops should be plentifully

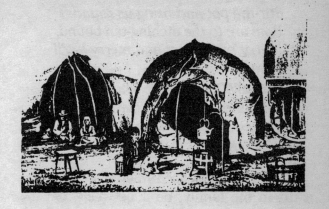

included. Stir the cookpot only clockwise, and when moving around it, move only clockwise. The stirring spoon must be a wooden one, and the cookpot must be iron.

On the fire over which the cookpot hangs, throw handfuls of cedar chips; and at some time during the cooking, sprinkle onto the fire three spoonfuls of salt.

Any time the pot is stirred, it must be stirred in batches of three, i.e., three, six, or nine clockwise stirs at a time. During these stirrings the mother will say:

Stir the pot and bring us round;
Rom are to the atching-tan bound.
Merry we'll meet and merry we'll
    part[3]
And merry will be the company
    found.

HEALING OLD WOUNDS

This is magick used when there has been
a rift in the family, be it between two individuals or between two whole groups
within the family. Once again it can be
recognized as basic sympathetic magick.

Take a long white candle and break it into
as many parts as there are factions. However,
be careful not to break the wick—only the wax.
On each section of the candle carve the name
of the individual or the initials of the major
figures in the dispute (i.e., should it be one whole
branch of the family against another, with
perhaps as many as 20 persons in each group,
then just mark the initials of the leaders,
such as the father and mother or grandmother).

Lay the broken candle on a sheet of
clean parchment (paper will do). Light a pink

---

[3]Wiccans may recognize this expression; they have the same one: "Merry
meet, merry part, and merry (may we) meet again."

(best), red (second best) or white (third choice) candle and hold it over the broken candle so that the melting wax drops down onto the breaks, sealing them. The broken candle should be slowly turned, keeping it on the parchment, so that all sides of the breaks become joined by the falling wax. As this is done, the magician should say "Heal! Heal! Heal!" repeating it as necessary until the white candle is whole again.

When the engraved candle is once again whole, stand it upright in a holder and light it. It should then be left to burn down completely.

TO BRING ABOUT THE RETURN OF A RUNAWAY

It is seldom that a Gypsy child will run away from home. Not so in the world of the gaujo. So it is not uncommon for a distraught mother to go to a Gypsy mother and ask how to cause the lost child to return. A popular, and reportedly successful, spell is as follows.

Take a handkerchief or article of clothing that belonged to the missing child. Place it on a table in front of you and lay a red rose on top of it. Say the following:

> Jelling *'cross the* pani,
> Jelling *down the* drom.
> Velling *home to find you,*
> *As you move along.*
> *Return, return, my* tikni (tikno—
>   masc.).
> *Return; come home to me.*
> Sutti *no more along the* drom
> *And we will happy be.*

Rough translation:

> *Traveling across the water,*
> *Traveling down the road.*
> *Coming home to find you.*
> *As you move along.*
> *Return, return, my child.*
> *Return; come home to me.*
> *Sleep no more along the road*
> *And we will happy be.*

Now lay a handkerchief or article of clothing of your own on top of the child's and the rose. Sprinkle wild marjoram (dried or fresh) over everything, followed by freshly drawn stream water. Repeat the verse and then lay the objects in the bottom of an empty drawer. The runaway child will come back to claim his or her belongings within 21 days, it is said.

It is here worth mentioning a custom I found in Essex, in the east of England, followed when a husband has abandoned the family. In order to bring him back the mother will take the baby, or youngest child, and pass him or her through a split ash tree sapling. This is supposed to cause the father to return.

TO END SIBLING RIVALRY

Even in Gypsy families two boys, especially when close in age, can become competitive. It's not often as bad with girls, though a boy and a girl can be abrasive. It can also become a problem when a new baby is born; frequently there is jealousy and rivalry on the part of the other child, or children. To cure this the Romani mother will frequently resort to magick.

Take an object from each of the children, one that has been well handled by them. This can be an article of clothing, a toy, a coin, or whatever. Place the objects together in a bowl and carry to a running stream.

Find a vine that is climbing up a tree and cut several short lengths from it. Also cut several short lengths from one of the tree's branches. Lay these pieces across the top of the bowl containing the articles belonging to the children.

With another small bowl or cup, scoop water out of the stream (going *with* the current) and pour the water over the gathered branches so that it falls into the bowl onto the items within. Do this with seven scoops of water, or until the bowl is filled. Say:

> *The vine clings to the tree*
> *And they grow in harmony.*
> *So let these children cling to one*
> *   another,*
> *And grow in strength.*

The articles should be left in the water-filled bowl for at least 24 hours.

TO WELCOME A NEW BABY

Romanis hold great respect for all life—human, animal, and vegetable. They only kill animals for food, never in sport. They never kill more than they need. Similarly, even with herbs, roots, and vegetables they will take only what is needed. They are never wasteful. It is little wonder, then, that a birth is heralded and there is much celebration. When a child is born it may or may not be baptized in a church. But it will certainly undergo a "baptism" within the tribe.

Some European Gypsies build a large fire at the entrance to the tent when a child is born (the child is born in a *bender*, or tent— never in the vardo). This fire is to keep away evil spirits. It is kept burning until the child has been baptized. This is not a common practice in England, although it can be found there in isolated areas. At the birth, the mother lets down her hair, believing that by doing so the birth will be easier.

Baptism of the child is sometimes by complete immersion in water into which herbs or grain have first been thrown. Sometimes it is by pouring water over the child, with the water running out of a bowl and first over the blade of a knife. The belief here is that the sharp edge of the knife blade will transfer to the water and serve as protection for the child. In both cases the water is cold, running water taken from a nearby stream.

Elwood Trigg points out that in the six-teenth century, records show that Gypsies who had their children baptized in churches frequently had the ritual performed a number of times. The feeling seems to have been that if this "magickal rite" was good for the child once, it would be even more beneficial a number of times!

The Romani child is given at least two names when baptized. This is to confuse any evil spirits, so that they won't know who the child really is. The child will generally be called by one name, with the other(s) remaining secret.

FOR PEACE AT SOMEONE'S DEATH

For Gypsies there is far more concern for the living than for the dead. Yet the Rom believe there must always be a family vigil prior to the death of a family member. After the death there will then be the funeral, which must be followed by a proper period of mourning.

English Gypsies belief that the owl is a harbinger of death. If they hear an owl hoot-

ing away in the distance, then it means someone close to them will die. If the owl is close
by, with its cries loud and clear, then the person who will die is distant.

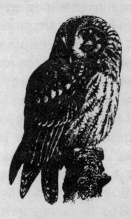

When an elderly member of the tribe is
ill, and certain that he or she is going to die,
word is sent out to all family members wher-
ever they happen to be scattered. They will
immediately return home, no matter from
how far, for this is the one event that takes
precedence over all others. The family members gather around the dying person's bed,
or outside around the tent or vardo. There is
always someone seated at the bedside until
the death. It is a time for much socializing,
with very little emotion shown regarding the

dying man or woman.

Once dead, the person is caught between the world of the living and the world of the dead. He or she will stay there until buried. In order to ease the stay there, and to prepare them for the transition to the world of the dead, there is a simple ritual that is sometimes performed by the shuvani (often without the knowledge of any of the other members of the tribe).

A small fire is lit—quite separate from any cooking fire—as soon as possible after the last breath. The fire should be laid carefully so that it can be started with one light and so that it will burn for a sufficient time without having to have more fuel added. Onto the fire are thrown thyme, sage, and rosemary, in that order. The dead person's name is chanted repeatedly as the shuvani walks backwards (widdershins, or counterclockwise) seven times around the fire, which is then left to burn itself out.

FAMILY UNITY

It is said that by throwing a small handful of salt on the family cooking fire every

Monday morning, you will keep the family together and help heal any rifts.

Another belief is that to roll a waggon wheel in a great circle around the outside of the vardo once a month at the New Moon will ensure family togetherness. It should be rolled clockwise.

One Gypsy woman in Norfolk assured me that the only sure way to keep the family together is to take a small clipping from every member's hair. These are then all placed together in a large leaf, which is rolled up and tied around with one of the mother's hairs. The package is then buried at the foot of an oak tree. The type of leaf in which the hair is wrapped was not specified, but it probably should be oak.

Togetherness can similarly be ensured by taking nail clippings from all family members and burying them at the foot of a tree—in this case a hawthorn or elm.

TO BRING UNDERSTANDING BETWEEN PARENT AND CHILD

This is a much-needed spell these days, it would seem. Though not so much with

Romani families, where there always seems
to be understanding between the children
and the parents.

To bring this understanding, first gather
seven long fronds of weeping willow (each at
least three feet in length). They should be cut
from the tree on the side closest to water.
Indeed, it is preferable that the tree be standing beside a river or stream, though this is
not essential. Lay the branches end to end in
a circle. No two cut ends should be together;
they should lay cut end against tip.

Holding an item of clothing belonging to
your child, stand in the center of this circle,
facing the east, and say:

> *Wisdom, love, and understanding*
> *Gather 'round us.*
> *Enclose us with your joy.*
> *Bring us together in all things;*
> *Making us as one.*

Lay the item of clothing on the ground,
in the center of the circle. Remove an article
of your own clothing and lay it on top. Then
starting in the east, gather up the branches of
willow one at a time and lay them on top of
the clothing. When they are all gathered and

piled, walk away without looking back. You may return after 24 hours to retrieve the clothing.

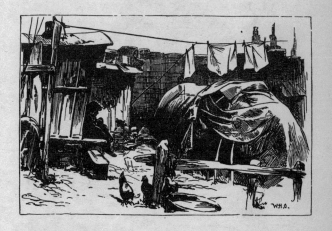

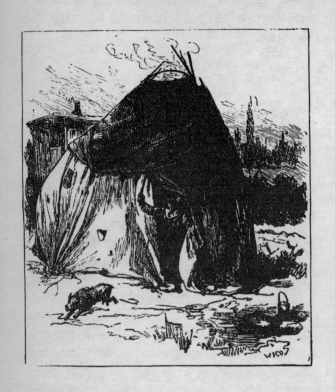

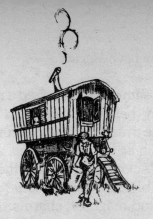

Gypsy Potions, Talismans, Amulets and Charms

Gypsies wear their wealth in the form of gold coins and jewelry. They don't trust banks (this also stems from the days when they were constantly traveling the roads, and banks were just not convenient for them). But along with the coins you can sometimes spot an unusual object hanging around a Romani neck—a talisman: a coin-size disc, square, or triangle with certain symbols engraved on it. It has been specially prepared and is worn for protection or to bring health, wealth, or love.

There was a time when Romani families would take their children to be baptized at the local church—and would keep going back to have the same child baptized a number of times! They believed there was a certain power in the ritual and would secrete various objects, such as buttons, stones, and coins, in the child's clothing. This way these objects would be blessed and become powerful talismans and magickal charms. This practice became so popular among Gypsies in sixteenth-century Germany that eventually the clergy refused to baptize Romani babies.

Once in a while the shuvani will give her customer a small package of herbs or a phial of liquid for discreet use in affairs of the heart. The Rom have a vast store of knowledge regarding herbs, roots, barks, flowers, and their uses. There are certain flora, they say, that can draw a man or a woman to you, and others that can cause anything from mild interest to raging desire. The Rom do not pass out these herbs indiscriminately. Nor do they give out the knowledge of where to find them, how to prepare them, or how to use them. Similarly, they do not casually pass out the secrets of their talismans and amulets.

My grandmother was much sought after for these "aids to love," both the herbal and the talismanic. She taught some of her knowledge to my mother (unfortunately, not everything), even though my mother was not Romani. From my mother, and from some of the older Gypsy women I have spoken with, I have managed to gather together a few "recipes."

LOVE SPRINKLES

When serving chicken (or *hotchi-witchi*, hedgehog, as the Rom do), sprinkle a little lovage (*Levisticum officinale*) over the portion to be served to your love ten minutes or so before it finishes cooking. This will increase his or her love for you and ensure faithfulness. It can similarly be sprinkled onto soup.

A secondary use for lovage is to sprinkle it in your bathwater. Soak in the tub for a while and you will find he/she is drawn to you almost as soon as you step out.

A little coriander dropped into a glass of hot mulled cider or hot wine will increase passion, the Gypsies say.

A teaspoonful of catnip herb (*Nepeta*

cataria) brewed in a cupful of water makes an excellent tea when sweetened with a little honey. Drunk by you and your lover just before going to bed, it will ensure warm "togetherness" through the night.

TO DRAW THE FULL POWER OF LOVE FROM YOUR PARTNER

In effect this is to overcome impotency or frigidity. Take equal parts of rosemary, lemon balm, and sage. Dry them, then grind them into powder. On the night of the New Moon, light a charcoal briquet and sprinkle the powder on as incense, and let it burn as you make love. As you lie together and the smoke rises, both of you say:

Herbs of love bring strength anew.
Let times of stress be very few.
Join two hearts and let love flow,
To consummate and end our woe.

Do this every night you make love until it is no longer necessary.

MAGICKAL VEGETABLES

There is a type of sympathetic magick performed by some shuvanis. They recommend the following for arousing a man for whom you are preparing a meal.

In the food you are preparing include carrots, parsnips, cucumbers and celery. These should never be cut crosswise into pieces but may be cut lengthwise. As you prepare these vegetables—wash and/or pare them—concentrate on your man and say the following spell:

> *Here is strength,*
> *Here is strength.*
> *Here is joy,*
> *Here is joy.*
> *Pleasure comes easily,*
> *Pleasure comes willingly,*
> *Pleasure comes!*

Repeat this seven times as you prepare the vegetables, all the time seeing your man as you would like him. It is said that this simple charm can cause a man to stop halfway through his meal and make passionate love to the cook!

ATTRACTION HERB

Along with the above recipe, it is said that if you put just a pinch of Bethroot in whatever you are cooking, the person to whom you serve it will be drawn to you in a very strong, romantic way.

Another way to draw your lover to you without using herbs is to obtain one of his or her shoes and keep it underneath your bed. This supposedly will draw the shoe's owner to that bed.

MANDRAKE MAGICK

The mandrake root has been considered magickal for centuries, because it grows naturally shaped like a human figure. The American mandrake (*Podophyllum peltatum*) is not related to the European variety (*Mandragora officinarum*, or *Atropa mandragora*) but all varieties *are poisonous*, so they should not be taken internally except under medical supervision.

Many Gypsies carry a piece of mandrake with them, either on their person or in

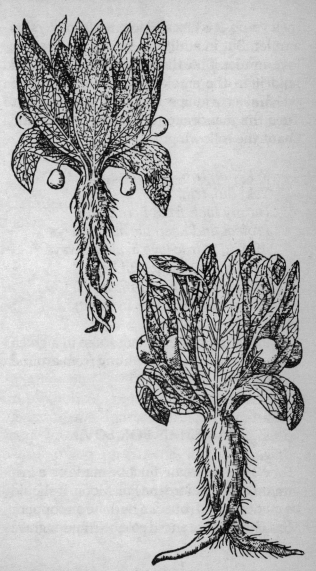

their vardo. It is first and foremost a protection amulet. But in addition, it can be a positive love amulet. Take the piece of mandrake and hold it in the smoke of a wood fire onto which alder or juniper twigs have been thrown. Turn the mandrake root in the smoke and chant the following:

> Yek, dui, trin, (one, two, three)
> Yek, dui, trin,
> Let my luck from here begin.
> Protect and keep me all my days
> And bring true love in all the ways.
> Let my heart so joyful be;
> Shoon, dick, te rig dré zi.
> (Hear, see, and bear in mind).

Place the piece of mandrake in a green silken bag, which can be hung from around the neck.

TALISMAN FOR LOVE

A love talisman must be made on a Friday, on or just before the Full Moon. It should be made on gold (but can be done on copper). Most Gypsies use an old gold coin and engrave over the impressions. Many seek out a really old coin that has been worn fairly smooth. You can use a proper engraving tool, though most Rom just sharpen a nail and use that. As you engrave, you must concentrate your thoughts on the one you love. This talisman will keep that love strong for as long as you both shall live. On the obverse, engrave the following:

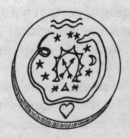

On the reverse engrave:

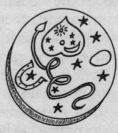

On the night of the Full Moon itself, wash the talisman in pure spring water (which can be easily obtained from a supermarket) and then hold it in the palm of your left hand. Breathe on it seven times, then hold it up high towards the Moon so that the light of the Moon shines on it. Say the name of your love aloud seven times. Then kiss the talisman and hang it around your neck.

LOVE BEADS

The wearing of certain natural beads in a necklace can act as a magickal love magnet. Acorns and sunflower seeds are good for this.

Collect the seeds, making sure they are clean and dry (if you want to make the necklace more attractive you can also add dried red and yellow corn kernels and melon seeds, interspersed). Soak the seeds in warm water for about an hour, then dry them thoroughly with paper towel. Use a sharp needle and doubled thread. A strong carpet thread is good for this. Push the needle through the fleshy end of any corn kernels and through the pointed end of melon seeds and sunflower seeds. Acorns need to be drilled first of all. This can be done simply enough by using an awl and pushing it through the midpoint of the nut.

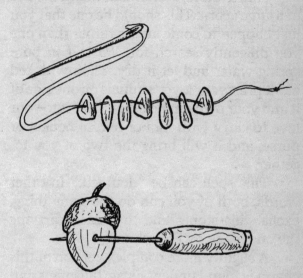

Coating the seeds with clear nail varnish will help preserve them.

Wearing a necklace of acorns or sunflower seeds will not only attract the opposite sex, it will also ensure fertility, so be warned!

LOVE PEBBLES

Find a round, white stone about the size of a large acorn. This should be one that you just happen to come across rather than one you diligently search for. Wash it in pure spring water and let it dry. Then with red paint print your lover's initials on one side of it and your own on the other. Give it to your love to carry with him or her, in pocket or purse, and it will bring the two of you together.

This spell can be "doubled." In other words, both of you can do the same thing, exchanging stones and then each carrying the one made by the other.

A slightly more complex version of this charm is found under Gypsy Talismans and Amulets on p. 117.

CARRY YOUR LUCK WITH YOU

Gypsies will carry a little five-finger grass, or cinquefoil (*Potentilla canadensis*), with them for luck. To have some in your pocket will make you lucky in love.

Bay leaves work much like five-finger grass. To carry a bay leaf is to carry luck. When you write a letter to your loved one, enclose a bay leaf in the envelope and it will increase their love for you.

Acorns are tokens of sexual love and desire. To have an acorn in your pocket when you meet with your love is to live dangerously! If you are feeling amorous, slip an acorn into your love's pocket without him or her seeing, and see what happens.

Lodestone is a natural magnet. It works for love. As with the acorns (above), carry a lodestone and slip a second one into your lover's pocket. They will draw you together.

Gypsies believe that if a woman sprinkles dried lavender (or passion flower) in a man's hatband, he will always think of her. (There is a similar charm whereby to sprinkle bracken in a man's hatband will make him cranky— not recommended!)

BIRTHING BITS

The Gypsies say that in cases of difficult childbirth one should lay a sharp axe underneath the bed. This will make the birth much easier.

It is important to always stir a cauldron clockwise, but this is especially important when the mother is giving birth. To stir it counterclockwise will make the birth very difficult.

A mother should let down her hair when giving birth, to make the birth easier.

When born, the baby should be immediately wrapped in a shirt belonging to the father. This will bring it luck, joy, and strength.

Charles Godfrey Leland, in *Gypsy Sorcery and Fortunetelling* (1891), states that when a Gypsy woman is with child "she will not, if she can help it, leave her tent in full moonshine. A child born at this time, it is believed, will make a happy marriage."

GYPSY POUCHES

Magickal pouches are found universally. Australian aboriginals, Amerindian shamans, Voodoo Bokos, African medicine men, European wisewomen—all employ pouches stuffed with various ingredients that they feel bring health, wealth, luck (good or bad), and/or protection. They may be called *wanga*, *gris-gris*, *mojo* bags, or whatever. The Gypsies, too, make and carry such items. Depending on the purpose, so do the contents vary. The name for a Gypsy pouch is *putsi*, the real meaning of which is "pocket."

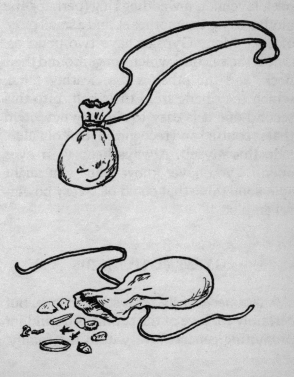

For love, the Romanis make little bags of red silk, which they fill with rose petals, acorns, a piece of amber, cinnamon, two cloves, a bean, a piece of orris root, and a silver or gold coin. This is worn next to the skin. Occasionally they use small chamois leather pouches rather than silk.

Some Gypsies also include such items as a small bird's feather, a piece of lemon peel, lavender, a wedding ring (perhaps the mother's or grandmother's), and a small piece of coal. Many Gypsies have two pouches. One is the silk one, which hangs around their neck, and the other is the leather putsi, which they hang from their belt. Into this second one it is easy to slip any new item that is spotted and recognized to be of value. I do this myself. Always keep your eyes open . . . you never know when you might spot something that could be a very powerful amulet.

GYPSY POTPOURRIS

Not necessarily for a specific love, but certainly for love of the countryside and for promoting general love within the family,

Romanis make use of potpourris in their vardos (they also make a great many to use for sales items). This is an ancient custom, again found all around the world, and tying in with the use of incenses.

There are actually two types of potpourri. The first is the small muslin bag that is filled with flowers or herbs and placed in drawers. The other is a mixture that is left out in an open dish to scent a room. Both have their uses. Potpourris may be very practical to the Gypsies, since many flower scents are useful in repelling insects and in keeping down mold and mildew.

Go out to gather your materials in the mid to late morning on a dry day. The Sun should have dried off the dew, yet not have grown strong enough to have diminished the strength of the fragrance. When gathering the flowers and leaves, never take bruised or damaged ones. Flowers are best picked just before they reach full bloom.

Drying what you have gathered is the most irksome part of the job. The flowers and leaves need to be laid out and spread evenly on sheets of paper in a cool, dry place. Spread them well so that they are not lumped or piled on top of one another (that leads to them turning brown and rotting). They have to be left there for about two weeks, turning them every day.

Here are recipes used by Romanis:

Mix together equal amounts of rose and lavender blossoms. Add as much rose geranium as you have of the rose and lavender together. Separately mix 2 oz ground cinnamon, 2 oz whole cloves, 1 oz cardamom seeds, 4 oz gum benzoin (a fixative), 4 oz ground orris root, and 6 lb of coarse salt. Take regular canning jars and pour in about an inch layer of this mixture. On top of it lay an inch of the flower mixture. Continue to alternate layers till the jar is full, pressing each layer down firmly with a flat piece of wood. Cap tightly. Continue with other jars. Then put them away for about three months to mature. They will then be ready for use.

• • •

Mix together equal amounts of geranium leaves, rose petals, and lemon verbena leaves. You can also add other flowers if you wish. For every pound of this mixture, add a half ounce each of cinnamon, cloves, ground orris root, gum storax and gum benzoin, 4 oz Barbados sugar, and 4 oz salt. Mix thoroughly and store in a large, open jar. Leave it for a week, stirring it every day. It may then be poured out into bowls for use.

• • •

To make a nice sachet, gather lavender by cutting about 12 inches of the stems with the flower heads on and tying them together in bunches. Store them with the flower heads hanging down (hang the bunches over a line of string) in a cool, dark place. When they have thoroughly dried out and the flowers are brittle, break the heads off the stems and pack them into small muslin bags, ready for use.

GYPSY TALISMANS AND AMULETS

A talisman is a manmade magickal object designed to promote health, wealth, love, protection, or similar objectives. An amulet is much the same except that it is a *natural* object (e.g., a rabbit's foot or a stone with a hole through it). These are, once again, magickal items that are found universally and that have been found in all ages, going back to the early caveman. The Gypsies have used talismans and amulets as long as they have been traveling. They make and use them both for themselves and for others.

Gypsy love tokens are much sought after in England. They are regarded as being especially potent. There is a tremendous variety of them, so I can detail only a few here.

Stone Talisman

This is almost a combination amulet and talisman, since it is a natural object that has been worked upon to give it its magickal properties.

Find a round, smooth stone about the size of a half dollar. If it is flattish, all the better. Wash it in clear well or stream water and let it dry. Then with paint, felt-tipped marker or nail varnish (a popular medium with modern-day Gypsies), mark on one side of it the initials or full names of the two lovers. On the other side draw the design shown:

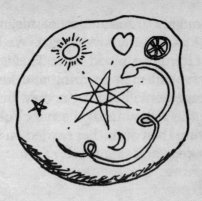

This should be done during the waxing cycle of the Moon. The design is an old traditional Gypsy design for love. At the Full Moon, go out into the open and lay the stone flat on the ground with the name side up. With a sharp *choori* (knife) cut your finger and allow a spot of blood to fall on the stone. Take the stone in the palm of your left hand, holding it up in the light of the Moon. After a few moments turn over the stone and repeat holding it up. In this way both sides will get "moon struck." Now take the stone in your right hand and hold it over your heart. Looking up at the Moon, say:

Mandi's ratti katé 'te mandi
piramni. Mendi dui si yek.

Roughly translated that means, "My blood I give to my sweetheart. We two are one." Literally a blood oath. This is a most powerful talisman to bring and keep you both together. The stone should be placed under the pillow until the next Full Moon and, from then on, either carried on the person or kept in a safe place.

Stone Amulets

Any stone having a natural hole through it is considered by the Romani to have great magickal power. It is referred to as a *daibar*, or "woman stone," much like the "hag stone" of Witchcraft. It is a very potent amulet both for luck and for protection, and especially for fertility. Farmers in Cumberland, England and surrounding areas still hang such stones around the necks of their cattle and from the byre, or barn, doors.

Similarly, long, round-section stones that are phallus-like are equally respected for their magickal fertility properties. Such stones can often be found on beaches (Brighton Beach is typical), and Gypsies can sometimes be seen moving slowly along the shorelines, searching for such fetishes. However, any found this way are usually sought in order to sell. The stone with true power is the one that you just "happen" to come across. This is the one that is kept by the Romani.

Horse Brasses

Horse brasses have been found throughout Europe for centuries and are still prominent in England. The originals were probably designed to reflect away the evil eye. Later they came to cover the keeping away of diseases and the promotion of fertility for the animals. One very interesting archaeological find, at Wilcote (Oxon.) in England, is a bronze bull's head dating from Roman times. It clearly shows a roundel on the animal's forehead—a talisman for the animal that pulled the plough in those days. Gypsy horses always wear horse brasses. When there are a number of brasses together on one strip of leather, it is called a martingale.

There is a tremendous range of designs (see p. 122). Perhaps the most popular is that of the Sun. This is displayed sometimes with the Sun's face in the center and sometimes with just the radiating rays. Almost as popular is the Moon, which is found in a variety of styles. There are designs with stars,

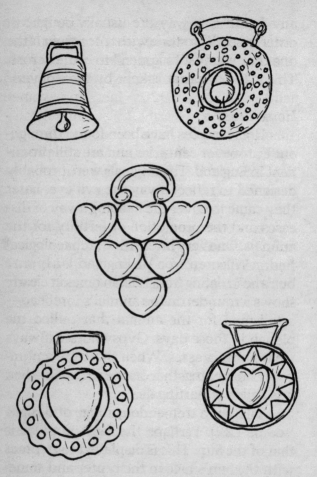

bells, anchors, animals, birds, flowers, hearts, and much more. From the point of view of love, the heart design is our interest in this book.

Many of the heart design horse brasses were actually to "give heart" to the animal that wore it, to give it strength. But they can be equally efficacious for love. In recent years (since the early 1920s) men and women have taken to wearing these animal talismans themselves—some for protection but many for love. They are generally heavy but can be effective hanging from a belt or, especially, worn as a belt buckle. It is not always easy to attach them to a belt, but it can be done utilizing the large press-studs used in leatherwork. Along with the various heart designs are a number of brasses with acorns on them. These can be good to wear to promote fertility and strength.

Coin Talismans

Gypsies have a fondness for gold coins, and particularly like wearing them as jewelry. This is because they were (and are), as nomads, unable—and certainly unwilling—to use banks to keep their money. What better way to carry their wealth than by adorning themselves? Gypsies wear gold necklaces and bracelets, and even gold fringing with small coins can be seen on their vests and other clothes. In addition to simply transporting their wealth, they also use coins for the making of talismans. Coins certainly are perfect for this, as regards size, material, and availability.

Various magickal texts have been available, to those who searched, for the past two or three hundred years or more. Ancient grimoires have passed from hand to hand across the length and breadth of Europe. The Gypsies certainly had a hand in this distribution. As bearers of arcane occult knowledge, they were in a position to recognize rare works of magick when they saw them. Although most Gypsies were illiterate and couldn't read the books, they were certainly able to recognize them from their illustrations. And many were familiar with the titles, if not the actual texts. A number of these grimoires dealt with the making of talismans, and pictured these as being circular, in the shape of coins. The easy way for the Gypsies to make such talismans, then, seemed to be to take a gold coin and engrave over the impression already on it. This is what the Gypsies did, and what they still do today.

If you don't have a gold coin, you can

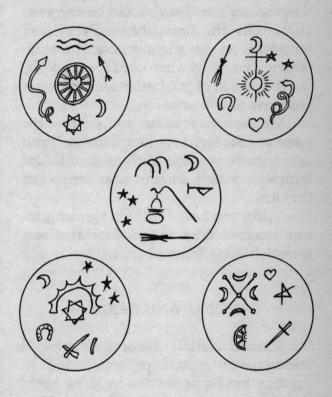

use copper. Copper discs are readily available at craft and hobby stores. Copper is the metal of Venus and is, therefore, appropriate for a love talisman.

On p. 125 are some typical Gypsy love talisman designs. They should be engraved on the coin/disc during the waxing cycle of the Moon. As you engrave, concentrate on putting your energies into what you are doing. See the person of your affections. Pour out your love to him or her.

On the reverse of the coin, engrave the name of your loved one and yourself. If you can, include symbols such as astrological birth signs or birth dates to make them more personal.

When you have finished engraving, repeat the dedication to the Moon that was given for Stone Talisman (p. 119).

STONES AND HERBS

There is a variety of superstitions found among the different Gypsy tribes concerning love and its promotion by using herbs and precious and semiprecious stones. Here are a few that I have found in my travels.

ACORN An ancient fertility/phallic symbol that shows up a lot in Romani lore.

AGATE If you place this stone on the left breast of a sleeping woman, when she awakes she will tell you truly whether or not she loves you.

AMBER Amber, along with jet, is worn a great deal by Gypsies. Amber is regarded as very much a panacea, being especially effective in affairs of the heart. If you hold a piece of amber up to the Full Moon and gaze through it, they say you will see the face of your true love.

AMBERGRIS This is a secretion from the intestines of the sperm whale and is an ingredient found in many perfumes. It is very potent in attracting a man to a woman. Interestingly enough, most momen do not care for it, but it certainly works "like a charm" on men!

AMETHYST Known mainly for its properties in curing drunkenness, amethyst is also a love token. It works on a woman much as ambergris (*see above*) does on men. A man who wears amethyst will find women attracted to him.

ANGELICA If you suspect that you are being attracted to someone magickally, against your wishes, then you can counteract the pull with angelica (*Angelica archangelica* or *Angelica sylvestris*). Simply place seven leaves of the plant in a small white silk pouch and hang it around your neck, suspended over your heart.

ASPARAGUS An aphrodisiac. Rather than the plant itself, take the roots and boil them in wine. Drink this for seven mornings in a row, with no breakfast. The Gypsies say it is a sure way to arouse lust.

BADGER A badger's foot is supposed to arouse passion. Keep it under your mattress at night; carry it in your pocket by day.

BEAN Beans have been regarded as potent sexual amulets for centuries in many different cultures. They are found in the Gypsy putsis (*see* p. 113) and are often carried loose in the pocket.

BERYL Recommended for renewing dying love between husband and wife, also for strengthening existing love. Wear it in a ring or necklace.

BLOODSTONE Known especially for easing childbirth. It also prevents miscarriage.

CARAWAY If you chew the caraway seed while thinking about the one you love, they will surely become yours.

CARROT Once thought to be a powerful aphrodisiac, when chopped finely and served in wine it can certainly put you in the right frame of mind for amorous pursuits.

CHALCEDONY "The one who wears it is lucky in love," say the Gypsies of Kent. It is also worn by nursing mothers to increase their milk.

CINNAMON A light sprinkling on just about any food will cause amorous thoughts. If used with discretion at the appropriate time, it can lead to an evening of delights.

CINQUEFOIL *(Potentilla canadensis)* Otherwise known as five-finger grass, it is a favorite for luck in general and certainly to be lucky in love.

CLOVES Fertility symbols, used in various love potions and as amulets.

COAL A piece of coal is a lucky amulet, sometimes applied to love. Sometimes found in putsis.

COCKEREL   The tail feathers of a cockerel are much sought after by Romanis as love amulets for men. They are said to draw a woman from miles away. Many a Gypsy Rom wears a cock's tail feather in his hat. A cock's comb was once supposed to be a powerful aphrodisiac.

CORIANDER   Seeds used in love potions.

CROW   An old English folk belief (not necessarily Gypsy) was that to bury a crow's eye under your bed would excite lust. Gypsies have great respect for crows and, more so, for ravens.

CUCUMBER   Another supposed aphrodisiac.

CYCLAMEN   The dried root, when crushed and mixed in with wine, is used as a love potion.

DOG   The dog *(jukkel)* is not "man's best friend" to the Gypsy; it is the horse (dogs are never allowed to enter a tent or vardo). But the dog is used a lot for hunting. The favorite breed is the lurcher—part greyhound, or whippet, and part sheepdog. There is an old love spell in which a sheet is thrown over a dog and a bitch when they are mating. If that sheet is later wrapped about a woman (or a man), she (he) will then willingly go to bed with you.

EEL An aphrodisiac. Jellied eels are a delicacy in many areas. An eel skin worn wrapped around the thigh will cure impotency.

ELDER Elder berries gathered on St. John's Eve are powerful love amulets. They can either be made into wine themselves or mixed with wine and given as a drink. Or they can be dried and carried as an amulet. An elder twig, cut in the light of the Full Moon and then cut into seven pieces, is another love amulet.

EMERALD If you suspect your lover of being unfaithful, wear an emerald and he (or she) will reveal himself.

FEATHER The feather of a small bird, particularly that of a wren or robin (English robins are much smaller than North American ones) are good love amulets (see also Cockerel).

FERN Seeds of the fern are used in love potions. However, there are both male and female ferns. You must use the seeds from a male fern for a potion to be taken by a female, and vice versa.

FOX The testicles of a fox, dried and powdered, are used as an aphrodisiac. The right testicle should be given to a woman, the left to a man.

FROG The bones of a frog that has been eaten and cleaned by ants are traditionally excellent love amulets.

GOAT To anoint one's loins with the semen of a he-goat is to prepare for a veritable orgy of sex! So say some of the Gypsies I have spoken with. Certainly the goat has always been historically regarded as an especially carnal, lustful beast. Powdered goat horn is supposed to be a great aphrodisiac. To carry a tuft of goat hair, especially taken from the tail, is a good love amulet.

HARE The genitals of a hare are used in potions to arouse lust.

HENBANE (*Hyoscyamus niger*) An ingredient in love potions. It should, however, be used (if at all) with extreme caution, since the whole plant is poisonous.

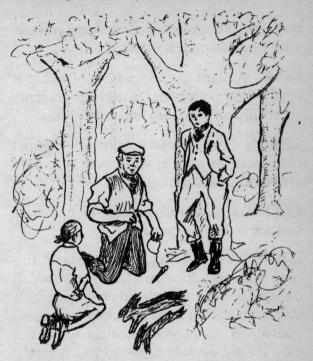

JASMINE (*Jasminum officinale*) It is said that the smell of just a few drops of jasmine oil will arouse the coldest man or woman. Mixing the oil with almond oil and massaging it into the body is supposed to cure frigidity and impotency.

JET With amber, the favorite stone of the Gypsies and used as a love amulet.

LAVENDER A gentle love awakener. Sprinkle

lavender under your lover's bed and you will soon be sharing it, they say!

LEEK   A plant in the onion family that is used in love potions in the north of England, especially in Yorkshire and Lancashire.

LEMON   The peel of the lemon, when grated finely and steeped in wine, is said to be a powerful sexual stimulant.

LETTUCE   Like leeks, used in love potions. Lettuce is also a soporific.

LODESTONE   A magickal love magnet, this magnetite will draw two lovers together. It can also be used to draw out one's feelings, if you or your lover have difficulty expressing yourselves. It is a great healing stone, but care should be taken not to use it in the vicinity of rubies or garnets, for it can damage these precious stones.

MANDRAKE   The European Mandrake (*Mandragora officinarum*) is not related to the American Mandrake (*Podophyllum peltatum*). Although the American variety has many useful medicinal qualities, it is the European version which has the traditional magickal properties. Both plants are poisonous if taken internally. Gypsies use the mandrake as a love amulet, among other things. They say it will ensure lasting love between couples if each carries a piece from the same plant.

MISTLETOE A centuries-old symbol for love. To kiss beneath the mistletoe is to set the seal on one's love. It will also ensure fidelity on the part of both partners.

MUSK A substance obtained especially from the small Asiatic deer, or musk deer. Worn by a man, it has the effect of drawing women to him. A powerful love potion.

MYRRH Used in incenses and oils to draw a lover to you.

NETTLE (*Urtica dioica*) The common stinging nettle is found in all parts of England and all over the United States. Fresh juice of nettle, or an infusion of it, will stimulate the flow of a nursing mother's milk. Young plants are sometimes used in love potions.

ORRIS ROOT (*Iris florentina*) A love amulet that is usually included in the Gypsy putsi. Carrying a piece of orris root can work in a similar way to mandrake root.

PIGEON   A white pigeon, or dove, seen flying from left to right across your path is a sign that you will shortly meet your true love.

RABBIT   A rabbit's foot is, of course, well known as a lucky charm. A hare's foot is more favored by Gypsies, but whether it is a rabbit's or a hare's, if from a white animal it is especially good for luck in love. Carry it with you in pocket or purse, hang it from your key ring, or wear it as a pendant.

ROSEMARY (*Rosmarinus officinalis*) A small linen bag filled with dried rosemary leaves and/or flowers, worn under your clothing and hanging over your genitals, will bring lovers to you in a hurry.

ROWAN (*Sorbus aucuparia*) Otherwise known as the European mountain ash, its berries are sometimes made into a necklace that is a good love amulet. Gypsies also frequently make the fruit into a jam, which is supposed to be a mild aphrodisiac.

RUBY   An excellent love amulet when worn in a ring.

ST. JOHN'S WORT (*Hypericum perforatum*)

When cut on St. John's Eve and carried next to the heart, this herb can be a powerful love amulet. The orange-yellow flowers are frequently pressed between the pages of a book and kept in the vardo as a general "heart center" for family love.

SNAIL Although probably not used today, it used to be that crushed snail shells were used in love potions. They were very highly regarded, with the stronger recipes reputedly invoking sexual desire and lust.

STRAW Straw dolls, "corn dollies," or "poppets" are very much used in love spells. (See p. 143—Cloth Dolls and Corn Dollies.)

TURQUOISE Worn by both lovers after a quarrel, this stone will bring the two back together again.

VERVAIN (*Verbena officinalis*) Long looked upon as an aphrodisiac, vervain is highly regarded by the Gypsies. It is best gathered on the first day of the New Moon, before sunrise. The dried flowers can be carried or kept under the pillow to bring luck and love.

HERBAL BATHS

Gypsies are really not heavily into bathing! There is good reason for this. With any nomadic people it will be found that there is a great appreciation of water. It is not always easy to come by and so must be used sparingly and with discretion. Never waste water on washing the body when it may be desperately needed for drinking.

But despite this, there are times when a bath must be taken, and times when it must not only be taken but must be taken in a certain manner . . . an herbal bath to promote affairs of the heart, for instance.

Romani women have one or two time-honored recipes for herbal baths, for those times when it is really important: to attract a love, to seal a lovers' contract, to repair a damaged love, for example. Here are the ones I was able to find.

1. Into your bath water drop rose petals and jasmine flowers, a small number of mint leaves, and some comfrey root. Let them steep there for at least five minutes, then you can either get into the bath immediately or pull the ingredients out first and then get in.

Most Romanis leave the herbs and flowers in with them.

2. Rosemary and carnation petals in equal parts plus half the amount of lavender. Add a sprinkling of fennel and thyme.

3. Mint, lavender, and marjoram steeped first, for at least five minutes. Then add a sprinkling of rose petals and a pinch of basil.

4. Prepare a pot of herbal tea beforehand. Use one teaspoonful each of rosemary, valerian, vervain, mint, and cinnamon. Let it steep for about ten minutes, then pour it into the bath water. Sprinkle on top about a half teaspoonful of lovage (dried and powdered).

5. Simmer a quarter cup of lavender and a quarter cup of rose petals in a quart of water for 15 minutes. Add to your bath water.

6. Simmer a quarter cup of hops and a quarter cup of marjoram in a quart of water for 20 minutes, then add to your bath water.

7. Simmer a quarter cup of peppermint and a quarter cup of linden flowers in a quart of water for 15 minutes, then add to your bath water.

Generally the above can be done with either fresh flowers/herbs or dried ones. While soaking in the bath, you should concentrate on your desire, be it to bring love, heal a rift, or consummate a union.

UNLUCKY DAYS

There are certain days throughout the year that many Gypsies believe are unlucky days for love. On these dates no one should try to sway another, bring any two people together, or—least of all—get married. These days are as follows:

January 1, 2, 6, 14, 27
February 1, 17, 19
March 11, 26
April 10, 27, 28
May 11, 12
June 19
July 18, 21
August 2, 26, 27
September 10, 18
October 6
November 6, 17
December 5, 14, 23

GYPSY BEAUTY SECRETS

Gypsy women are some of the most beautiful women in the world. How do they get that way? Are they born beautiful? Many are, yes, but not all. And for those who are not, there are some closely kept beauty secrets.

To wash your face with dew every morning is believed to keep the complexion clear. Rain water also has been used, but these days of acid rain give one pause for thought.

If you have very dry hair, warm some olive oil and apply it to the hair, using cotton balls. Work slowly over the head, working the oil in and being careful to cover the ends of the hair with the oil. Then dip a towel in hot water, wring it out, and wrap it around your hair. When the towel has cooled, reheat it and wrap it around again. Do this for a total of an hour, then thoroughly shampoo the hair.

A Gypsy skin freshener is made up of one part malt vinegar (apple cider vinegar will do) to eight parts of water. This is also good as a hair rinse.

A favorite Romani facial is a mixture of one egg with one tablespoonful each of honey and of milk. Beaten together, this is applied to the face and neck and left on for a period of ten to fifteen minutes before being washed off with warm water followed by cold water.

For men, tea made from wild cherry bark is an excellent hair tonic and hair restorer. A strong mixture worked into the scalp over a period of time is said to grow hair on a bald man.

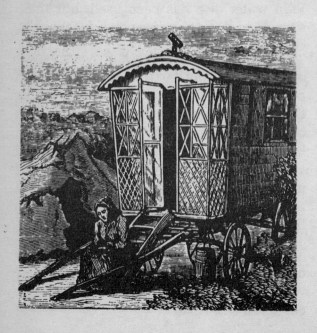

A tea made from sage is not only a good hair dressing but will also bring back the hair's natural color when it is starting to grey.

Some Romani women will take a lock of their hair and bury it at the foot of a willow tree. This is said to promote luxuriant growth, making the hair glossy and attractive.

If you cut your hair at the New Moon it will grow rapidly and richly. If you cut it in the waning cycle, it will grow very slowly.

Many a Romani woman will never brush her hair in artificial light. She will either do it in the daylight or will sit outside and do it in the light of the Moon.

CLOTH DOLLS AND CORN DOLLIES

Image magick is practiced worldwide. From the ancient Egyptians to present-day Voodooists, doll-like figures have been, and still are, made to represent a person and then affected magickally. The Gypsies certainly make use of this same magick. It is perhaps one of the oldest forms known, if not *the* oldest.

The basic idea is that if you make a

figure to represent a person, and name it (in effect, baptize it) for that person, then anything you do to that figure will be the same as actually doing it to the person it represents. If, for example, you make a cloth doll image of your lover and another of yourself, then bind the two of them together, you will cause the (real) two of you to bind together. Following the mandate that you must not interfere with another's free will, this would only be done with the consent of both parties, or by the two of you working together.

But let's look at the corn dollies first. There are many different types found in different parts of the country. For instance: the Suffolk Horn, the Essex Teret, the Mother Earth, the Vale of Pickering, and the Norfolk Lantern. Some tribes/individuals favor one style, some another. I will detail how some of these are made and then give more details on their actual use.

● ● ●

English corn is not the same thing as American corn, or maize, of the corn-on-the-cob variety. It is a hollow-stemmed form—a straw with a head much like wheat. Indeed, wheat (the more modern hollow straw, rather than the older pithy-centered variety), rye, and oats are also suitable for doll making, though barley is not. Collect some of the straw when nearly ripe, when the first joint below the ear is still green. If it is used within a week of being collected you won't need to dampen it. Once collected, if you are not going to use it right away, dry it in the sun (or even in a very slow oven, with the door open). Once dried it can be stored in boxes for years, if necessary, till needed.

The straw needs to be trimmed by cutting it off at the top, above the top joint and just below the ear, and at the bottom just above the bottom joint. There is invariably a leaf that grows out from either the bottom or second joint. This should be removed.

If dried, start out by laying a bundle of straws in a long dish, or stand them upright in a tall vase, and pour boiling water over them. Or you can hold them with tongs, over a bucket, and pour the water over them. Then take them and roll them in a damp cloth to keep them soft and supple and easy to work with.

Pick out five good length straws, of about equal length, and tie the ends tightly together with thread. With the short ends held tightly in your left hand, bend four of the straws down at right angles, then bend the fifth (center) one down so that it is on top of straw #1 (see figure 1).

Now, taking straw #1, move it under straw #5 and towards straw #4 (see figure 2). Then bend straw #1 up and over straw #5 so that it now lies alongside straw #2 (figure 3). Holding these two straws (#1 and #2) together, rotate the whole figure, clockwise, one place so that you are back where you started in figure 1. Now repeat the above action, only this time you will be moving straw #2 down towards #5, then up to be beside #3. Rotate again and continue. In other words, each time you start with a straw to the right, alongside another. The lower one of these two is swung to the bottom then bent up and over to lay beside the one at the top. Rotate and start again. In this way you will see that a definite shape comes into being (figure 4)—a spiral of square section.

The size of the square section can be determined and varied. You can place an object, such as a straight stick, in the center and work around it to fill it out. In making these dollies for magickal purposes it is com-

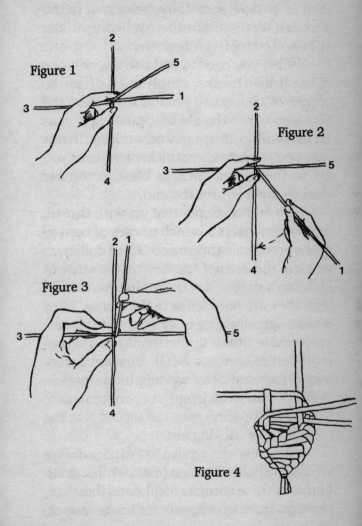

Figure 1

Figure 2

Figure 3

Figure 4

mon to enclose something belonging to the person it represents inside; a rolled-up diklo, or handkerchief, is a favorite.

When you need to add a straw, or if one of the straws breaks, simply cut it off at the corner of the square section and insert the new straw into the old one, pushing it in as far as it will go, then carry on working. In this way you can introduce thicker straws as you get to the center, then go back to thinner ones to taper off for the end.

The end is simply tied up with thread, or you can insert a bunch of ears of corn to give a head/hair appearance. Corn dollies, as you can see, are not "dollies" in the sense of children's dolls. They do not have arms and legs; they are not lifelike in that sense. They were originally simply symbols of the harvest used in rituals to give thanks and to promote future harvests. But if you want a more lifelike appearance for working image magick, then you can work lengths of corn crosswise through the figure, near the top, to give the idea of arms sticking out.

The American equivalent of corn dollies would probably be corn (maize) husk dolls. Certainly these are more lifelike and therefore, perhaps, more appropriate for image magick.

These can be easily made. You will need about 15 corn husks for a woman, about 12 for a man. Collect the husks and dry them in the sun, as above. Soak in hot water to make them pliable for use.

For the arms, tightly roll three husks approximately 2" x 5" and tie the ends with stout thread (figure 5). For the heads, roll scraps of husks into a ball about ¾" in diameter. Take two lengths of husk about 6" long by 1½" wide and place the ball in the center. Pull the husks around the ball and down to tie below (figure 6), then repeat with two more lengths the same size.

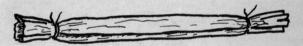

Figure 5

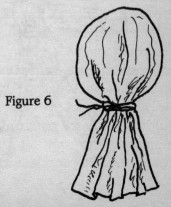

Figure 6

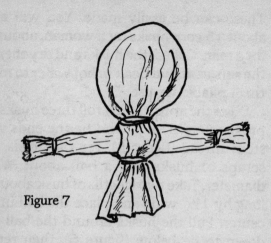

Figure 7

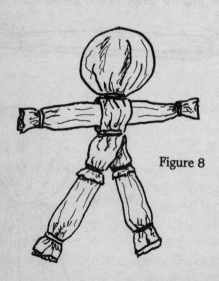

Figure 8

For the body, stick the arms through the hanging husks and tie at the neck and below the arms (figure 7). Now two types of body can be done: male and female.

(a) Male: Roll three husks, 3" x 5", stick half the hanging down husk into one end and tie around with thread. Do this again for the second leg (figure 8).

(b) Female: Use four to eight husks and group around the waist section, tying tightly with thread (figure 9). A shawl can also be added to this figure if desired. Wrap two husks 4"x 1½", folded and placed around neck then down, and crossed over chest, and tied (figure 10).

Cloth figures, sometimes called poppets, are equally easy. Gypsies use material from the person the figure will represent: cloth cut from a diklo, shirt, undershirt, skirt, or whatever. Consequently they are frequently of colored and patterned material rather than plain.

Folding the material in half, cut out two identical shapes (figure 11). Sew around the edges, leaving the top of the head open for

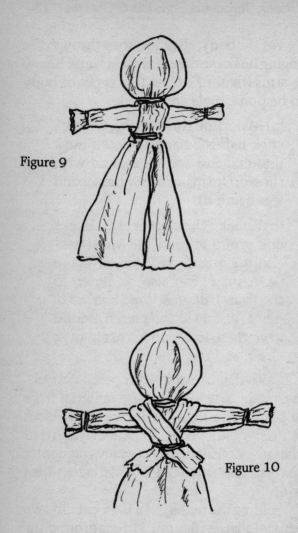

Figure 9

Figure 10

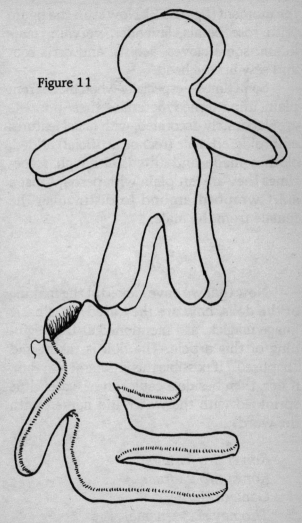

Figure 11

Figure 12

the moment (figure 12). Now stuff the figure with rose petals, lavender, vervain, marjoram, some cloves, acorns, and orris root and sew up the head.

Sometimes—especially when made from plain, unpatterned material—these poppets are elaborately decorated, with facial features embroidered, hair (real or artificial) added, clothes made and fitted, although sometimes they are left plain with perhaps just a skirt wrapped around to distinguish the female from the male.

• • •

Now that we have looked at the making of the dolls, how are they used? It is basic image magick, as I mentioned at the beginning of this article. The doll is taken and "baptized." If possible this is done at a stream; if not, then beside a cauldron of water. It is sprinkled with the water and named with the words:

Kon si tiro mamus?
Kon si tiro dadrus?
Gana ta Herne.
Tiro nav si . . . (name) . . . ;

Muk les si
Ta jel 'sa Duvvel[4].

("Who is your mother?
Who is your father?
Gana and Herne.
Your name is . . . . . ;
Let it be so
And go with God.")

In the example I used at the beginning of this article, there would be two poppets so named, one for each of the lovers, and they would then be placed together—perhaps even tied together with red ribbon[5]. Words would be said to the effect that the two people would cling to one another for always. Then they would be put away in some safe place.

Using just one figure—and here it could well be a corn dolly—the same baptism is undergone. Then the figure is told that it will do whatever is expected of it: be faithful to husband or wife, regain its virility, work at better understanding the spouse, etc. This is

---

[4] *Duvvel* is the Romani word for "God." Interestingly enough, with a Romani family in the southwest of England I found reference, in this verse, to *Duvveli—i* is the feminine ending.

[5] See *Buckland's Complete Book of Witchcraft* for details of a Wiccan poppet ritual for lovers that is similar to this.

usually done by the very person the figure represents; in other words you are doing the magick to achieve your own particular goal(s). This exemplifies the idea of not interfering with the free will of others.

Cloth dolls and corn dollies were once used a lot, especially by shuvanis, but they are seldom found today.

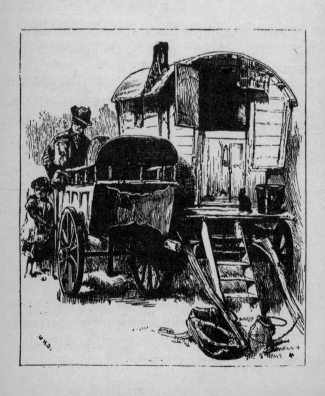

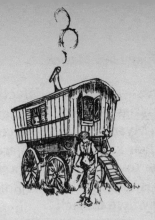

Breaking Camp

The beautifully kept horses tug at the shafts and proudly move the Gypsies' homes. The boxes and chicken baskets hanging underneath the waggons swing and sway as the brightly painted vardos cross the field and turn onto the road. The waggons start to head out, away from the village. Children run alongside, laughing and shouting. The campfires have been extinguished and the fields have been left neat and clean so that the Gypsies will be welcomed again next time they are in the area.

Once again the faces at the windows of the village peer out from behind curtains. But now there is a knowing smile on many of those faces—a glint of satisfaction of things taught, things learned. The Keepers of the Ancient Mysteries have once again dispensed their knowledge and are moving on to another town, where others eagerly await them. This is the path of the Romani. This is the Gypsy love magick.

Kushti bok
Raymond Buckland

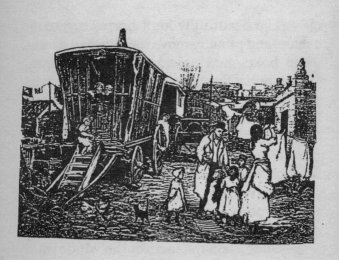

Note: The typical Gypsy vardo is a one-roomed waggon on four high wheels. The entrance is at the front, between the shafts, so that those inside can talk with the driver as they travel along. There is built-in furniture which includes beds, wardrobe, closets, cooking stove, table, chest of drawers, china closet, and bracket lamps. Underneath the vardo are many hooks for hanging pots, pans, baskets, and boxes. At the rear, underneath, is a built-in cupboard known as the kettle-box, where all the sooty cooking utensils used on the campfire are kept. The vardos are elegantly decorated both inside and out, their furnishings often featuring elegant Crown Derby china, lace trimmings, velvet drapes, polished mahogany, etched mirrors, and highly polished ornamental brasswork. *The Gypsies, Waggon-time and After*, by Denis Harvey (Batsford, London, 1984) and *The English Gypsy Caravan*, by C. H. Ward-Jackson and Denis E. Harvey (David & Charles, Devon, 1972) are two excellent books on the Romani homes.

STAY IN TOUCH

On the following pages you will find some of the books now available on related subjects. Your book dealer stocks most of these and will stock new titles in the Llewellyn series as they become available. We urge your patronage.

To obtain our full catalog write for our bimonthly news magazine/catalog, *Llewellyn's New Worlds of Mind and Spirit*. A sample copy is free, and it will continue coming to you at no cost as long as you are an active mail customer. Or you may subscribe for just $10.00 in the U.S.A. and Canada ($20.00 overseas, first class mail). Many bookstores also have *New Worlds* available to their customers. Ask for it.

Llewellyn's New Worlds of Mind and Spirit
P.O. Box 64383-053, St. Paul, MN 55164-0383, U.S.A.

TO ORDER BOOKS AND TAPES

If your book dealer does not have the books described, you may order them directly from the publisher by sending full price in U.S. funds, plus $3.00 for postage and handling for orders *under* $10.00; $4.00 for orders *over* $10.00. There are no postage and handling charges for orders over $50.00. Postage and handling rates are subject to change. We ship UPS whenever possible. Delivery guaranteed. Provide your street address as UPS does not deliver to P.O. Boxes. UPS to Canada requires a $50.00 minimum order. Allow 4-6 weeks for delivery. Orders outside the U.S.A. and Canada: Airmail—add retail price of book; add $5.00 for each non-book item (tapes, etc.); add $1.00 per item for surface mail. Mail orders to:

LLEWELLYN PUBLICATIONS
P.O. Box 64383-053, St. Paul, MN 55164-0383,
U.S.A.

Prices subject to change without notice.

SECRETS OF GYPSY DREAM READING
by Raymond Buckland, Ph.D.

The Gypsies have carried their arcane wisdom and time-tested methods of dream interpretation around the world. Now, in *Secrets of Gypsy Dream Reading*, Raymond Buckland, a descendant of the Romani Gypsies, reveals these fascinating methods.

Learn how to accurately interpret dreams, dream the future, dream for profit, remember your dreams more clearly, and willfully direct your dreams. The Gypsies' observations on dreaming are extremely perceptive and enlightening. They say that dreams are messages, giving advice on what is most beneficial for you. Many times these messages could mean the difference between happiness and misery—if not life and death.

In today's fast-paced, often superficial world, we need to listen to the Gypsies' words of wisdom more than ever. Listen to your dreams and achieve success, riches, better health—and more—in your waking hours!

0-87542-086-9, 224 pgs., mass market, illus. $3.95

BUCKLAND'S
COMPLETE GYPSY FORTUNE TELLER
by Raymond Buckland

This Llewellyn kit comprises a complete system of gypsy divination that everyone can explore and enjoy. It includes Ray Buckland's popular book, *Secrets of Gypsy Fortunetelling,* and *The Buckland Gypsy Fortunetelling Deck,* a beautiful 74-card deck which includes a distinctive Romani Major Arcana and a Minor Arcana composed of a regular poker deck and a handy 18" x 24" four color layout sheet. The two sides of the sheet illustrate different layouts—the Seven Star layout and the Romani Star layout. You can discover future events, hopes, fears, strengths and much more.

With *Buckland's Complete Gypsy Fortune Teller*, this time-honored system of divination is presented for the first time in a convenient and eminently usable format.

0-87542-055-9, book, 74-card deck, layout sheet $19.95

Prices subject to change without notice.

PRACTICAL COLOR MAGICK
by Raymond Buckland, Ph. D.

The world is a rainbow of color, a symphony of vibration. We have left the Newtonian idea of the world as being made of large mechanical units, and now know it as a strange chaos of vibrations ordered by our senses, but, our senses are limited and designed by Nature to give us access to only those vibratory emanations we need for survival.

> Learn the secret meanings of color.
> Use color to change the energy centers of your body.
> Heal yourself and others through light radiation.
> Discover the hidden aspects of your personality through color.

This book will teach all the powers of light and more! You'll learn new forms of expression of your innermost self, new ways of relating to others with the secret languages of light and color. Put true color back into your life with the rich spectrum of ideas and practical magical formulas from Practical Color Magick!

0-87542-047-6, 160 pgs., 5¼ x 8, illus., softcover $6.95

PRACTICAL CANDLEBURNING RITUALS
by Raymond Buckland, Ph. D.

Another book in Llewellyn's Practical Magick series. Magick is a way in which to apply the full range of your hidden psychic powers to the problems we all face in daily life. We know that normally we use only 5% of our total powers—Magick taps powers from deep inside our psyche where we are in contact with the Universe's limitless resources.

Magick need not be complex—it can be as simple as using a few candles to focus your mind, a simple ritual to give direction to your desire, a few words to give expression to your wish.

This book shows you how easy it can be. Here is Magick for fun, Magick as a Craft, Magick for Success, Love, Luck, Money, Marriage, Healing; Magick to stop slander, to learn truth, to heal an unhappy marriage, to overcome a bad habit, to break up a love affair, etc.

Magick—with nothing fancier than ordinary candles, and the 28 rituals in this book (given in both Christian and Old Religion versions)—can transform your life. Illustrated.

0-87542-048-06, 200 pgs, 5¼ x 8, softcover $6.95

**BUCKLAND'S
COMPLETE GYPSY FORTUNE TELLER
by Raymond Buckland**
This Llewellyn kit comprises a complete system of gypsy
divination that everyone can explore and enjoy. It includes
Ray Buckland's popular book, *Secrets of Gypsy Fortunetelling*, and *The Buckland Gypsy Fortunetelling Deck*, a beautiful
74-card deck which includes a distinctive Romani Major
Arcana and a Minor Arcana composed of a regular poker
deck and a handy 18" x 24" four color layout sheet. The two
sides of the sheet illustrate different layouts—the Seven
Star layout and the Romani Star layout. You can discover
future evaents, hopes, fears, strenths and much more.

With *Buckland's Complete Gypsy Fortune Teller*, this time-
honored system of divination is presented for the first time
in a convenient and eminently usable format.
0–87542–055–9, book, 74-card deck, layout sheet $19.95

**EARTH POWER:
TECHNIQUES OF NATURAL MAGIC
by Scott Cunningham**
Magick is the art of working with the forces of Nature to
bring about necessary, and desired, changes. The forces of
Nature—expressed through Earth, Air, Fire and Water—
are our "spiritual ancestors" who paved the way for our
emergence from the pre-historic seas of creation. Attuning
to, and working with these energies in magick not only
lends you the power to affect changes in your life, it also allows you to sense your own place in the larger scheme of
Nature. Using the "Old Ways" enables you to live a better
life, and to deepen your understanding of the world about
you. The tools and powers of magick are around you, wait-
ing to be grasped and utilized. This book gives you the
means to put Magick into your life, shows you how to
make and use the tools, and gives you spells for every purpose.
0–87542–121–0, 176 pgs., 5¼ x 8, illus., softcover $8.95